# SPECIAL SKILLS
# AND
# TECHNIQUES

# SPECIAL SKILLS
# AND
# TECHNIQUES

## Gretchen Beal Van Boemel, PhD, COMT

Doheny Eye Institute
University of Southern California
Department of Ophthalmology
Los Angeles, California

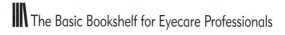 The Basic Bookshelf for Eyecare Professionals

*Series Editors* Janice K. Ledford, COMT • Ken Daniels, OD • Robert Campbell, MD

 6900 Grove Road, Thorofare, NJ 08086

Publisher: John H. Bond
Editorial Director: Amy E. Drummond
Assistant Editor: Lauren E. Biddle

Van Boemel, Gretchen B.
    Special skills and techniques / Gretchen Van Boemel.
        p. cm. -- (The basic bookshelf for eyecare professionals)
    Includes bibliographical references and index.
    ISBN 1-55642-349-7 (alk. paper)
    1. Eye-- Diseases-- Diagnosis. 2. Ophthalmic assistants.
    I. Title. II. Series.
        [DNLM: 1. Diagnostic Techniques, Ophthalmological.  WW 141 V217s 1999]
    RE76.V36  1999
    617.7'15--dc21
    DNLM/DLC
    for Library of Congress                                                    98-54626
                                                                                    CIP

Published by:        SLACK Incorporated
                     6900 Grove Road
                     Thorofare, NJ 08086-9447 USA
                     Telephone: 609-848-1000
                                856-848-1000
                     Fax: 609-853-5991
                          856-853-5991
                     World Wide Web: www.slackinc.com

Contact SLACK Incorporated for more information about other books in this field or about the availability of our books from distributors outside the United States.

Authorization to photocopy items for internal or personal use, or the internal or personal use of specific clients, is granted by SLACK Incorporated, provided that the appropriate fee is paid directly to Copyright Clearance Center, 222 Rosewood Drive, Danvers, MA 01923 USA, 978-750-8400. Prior to photocopying items for educational classroom use, please contact the CCC at the address above. Please reference Account Number 9106324 for SLACK Incorporated's Professional Book Division.

For further information on CCC, check CCC Online at the following address: http://www.copyright.com.

Last digit is print number: 10  9  8  7  6  5  4  3  2  1

# Dedication

To Jerry, Muffy, and Lynn.
Thank you for all of the love, encouragement, and inspiration you have given me.

# Contents

Exophthalmometry
    *by Barbara S. McLaughlin, COMT, and Gretchen Beal Van Boemel, PhD, COMT*
Pachymetry
Photokeratoscopy
Corneal Topography
Pupillometry
Pupillography
Ophthalmoscopy
    *by Barbara S. McLaughlin, COMT, and Gretchen Beal Van Boemel, PhD, COMT*

Overview of Psychophysical Testing
Advanced Color Vision Testing
Dark Adaptometry
The Macular Photostress Test
The Potential Acuity Meter
The Glare Test and the Brightness Acuity Test
Contrast Sensitivity

Overview
Ocular Microbiology
Identification of the Infectious Antigen
The Immune System

Axial Eye Length
Techniques of Axial Eye Length A-Scans
Brief Review
Probe Placement
Axial Eye Length Echo Patterns
Calculating Axial Eye Lengths with the A-Scan Echo Patterns
Conducting an Axial Eye Length Examination
IOL Power Calculations

# Acknowledgments

There are so many people who either directly or indirectly helped make this book possible. This book represents an accumulation of experiences I have had working in the field of ophthalmology over the past 17 years. I would like to first thank my mentor and friend, Thomas E. Ogden, MD, PhD, for taking a chance by hiring a new college graduate who had no experience in the field of ophthalmology and turning her into an electrophysiology technician. Thanks also to his wife, Carla, who taught me the nuts-and-bolts of ocular electrophysiology.

Deidre Martin inspired me to teach electrophysiology courses to technicians at the annual JCAHPO meeting and was always there to lend support and expertise. After my first course for JCAHPO, Fran Schoen and Alice Gelinas encouraged me to keep coming back. Thanks to both of them for their continued support. Thanks, too, to Juan Jimenez, MD, who encouraged me to write my very first book chapter many years ago.

Many individuals helped me learn other aspects of ophthalmology outside of the area of electrophysiology. Thank you to Melvin Trousdale, PhD, and Narsing Rao, MD, for allowing me to traipse through their microbiology and pathology laboratories, and learn about cells and microorganisms. Ronald Green, MD, has always encouraged my questions and was a tremendous help in the writing of the Ultrasonography section of this book. A. Frances Walonker, CO, COMT, single-handedly taught me everything there is to know about the technological aspects of ophthalmology, thus insuring that I could write about many of them with first-hand knowledge. I want to also thank Stephen Ryan, MD, and Ronald Smith, MD, former and current chairmen of the Department of Ophthalmology at the University of Southern California. Both of them have encouraged me to learn as much about and do as much within the field of ophthalmology as I possibly could. Thanks to John Irvine, MD, who helped maintain my sense of humor throughout the process of writing this book. Without the help of all of these people I could not have learned to love the field of ophthalmology as much as I do.

I would be remiss if I did not thank my major professor, Roxane Cohen Silver, PhD, who helped me learn how to keep on track even with a task that seems impossible to complete. Thanks also to my dear friend, Lynn Fowler, who helped me become a better writer by giving me bits of helpful criticism. Thanks to all of my family and friends who have not seen much of me over the past 2 years, but who have always been very understanding about my absence. Finally, I could not have completed this book without the clerical support of Wilma McConnell, the photographic support of Tracy Nichols and Nilo Davila, and the research support of Marissa Kattah, MD. My sincerest thanks go to my publisher and the editors at SLACK Incorporated, with a special thank you to Jan Ledford. I am truly grateful for all of your support.

# About the Author

Gretchen Beal Van Boemel, PhD, COMT, has worked in the field of ophthalmology since 1982. She received her undergraduate degree from California State University, Long Beach in the field of research psychology. After 1 year of working as a research assistant in the Department of Cardiology at the University of Southern California, Gretchen started working for the Doheny Eye Institute. She started out as a trainee in electrophysiology under the direction of Thomas E. Ogden, MD, PhD. Within several years, she was teaching electrophysiology courses to University of Southern California medical students and ophthalmology residents. She taught her first JCAHPO course on electrophysiology in 1985, and has taught various courses to ophthalmic technicians and registered nurses since that time. After 5 years she began teaching the practical aspects of ocular electrophysiology and psychophysiology to ophthalmology and psychology fellows (including foreign fellows).

After several years of working at Doheny, she found that she was fascinated by other facets of the field of ophthalmology. She first studied for her COT, and received it in 1985. Later she went on for her COMT certification, which she received in 1991. While at the Doheny Eye Institute, Gretchen also conducted original research in the areas of the usefulness of electrophysiology in the evaluation of the traumatized eye, and VER testing for unexplained vision loss. While conducting the later study, she became intrigued with what appeared to be psychogenic blindness in certain refugee women. With the assistance of a colleague specializing in psychology, Gretchen embarked on a research agenda that included investigating the consequences of severe trauma as the likely cause of psychogenic blindness in a group of older Cambodian women. That work resulted in national and international attention with appearances on ABC's *20/20* news program, a CNN evening news segment, British and German equivalents of *20/20*, as well as being featured in numerous newspaper articles, including a feature story in the *New York Times Magazine*.

As a result, Gretchen felt it necessary to continue her education, and she went back to graduate school while maintaining a full-time position as director of the electrophysiology and psychophysiology department at Doheny. She received her doctorate in Social Ecology with an emphasis in Health Psychology from the University of California, Irvine, in 1995.

Since receiving her doctorate, Gretchen has continued to work as director of the electrophysiology and psychophysiology department, but has taken on new responsibilities as well. She was asked to create a multidisciplinary low vision rehabilitation program that she currently heads. She is also the director of the Continuing Medical Education program at the Doheny Eye Institute. She has coordinated a grant on why preventable blindness occurs in diabetes and is currently investigating barriers to low vision care. Additionally, she has been a principal investigator on a Social Security Administration project aimed at assisting low income blind and visually impaired individuals in receiving appropriate benefits. She continues teaching JCAHPO courses, as well as courses at USC and California State University, Long Beach in the Health Science Department.

Gretchen truly loves the field of ophthalmology. It is her sincere hope that many of you will develop a greater appreciation of the field after reading this book. The areas covered are often considered tedious to get through, but she hopes that the case examples she has provided will allow these subjects to "come alive."

# Foreword

Most of my colleagues will agree with me when I say that a well-trained and knowledgeable technician is a tremendous asset to any ophthalmic practice. I have come to depend on my technicians and find their assistance invaluable. I have worked with individuals who have gone through college programs, as well as those who have been taught on-the-job. For the most part, there are few discrepancies between those who have been formally educated and those who have learned on-the-job, with the exception of understanding special diagnostic techniques in ophthalmology. The training programs usually cover these topics, but those who are job trained are limited to the expectations of their employers. If an employer has no need for a technician to learn to do an ERG, then the individual will not have the opportunity to learn about this test. For the COT® who has learned on-the-job, the challenge of taking the COMT® exam may come from having insufficient training in the specialized fields of ophthalmology such as microbiology, ultrasonography, electrophysiology, and psychophysical testing. With the publication of this book, the barrier to continued advancement in the field of ophthalmic assisting is lifted.

Gretchen Van Boemel, who herself was trained on-the-job, has taken several areas of ophthalmology that are not routinely covered in ophthalmic assisting books and has covered them well. The chapters are thorough and readable. She truly loves teaching, and loves the various special testing fields, especially ocular electrophysiology, and this shows in her writing.

This book will serve well as an introductory text for those attempting the COMT examination. Special testing techniques covered on the COMT examination are well detailed in this volume. For others, this book will serve as an excellent review source. I suspect that medical students going through an ophthalmology rotation will find this text an excellent overview of special testing techniques in ophthalmology. I am certain that some ophthalmologists who like Gretchen's teaching style, will find this a useful book for review as well. Gretchen Van Boemel has crafted a comprehensive textbook on special testing techniques in ophthalmology, a book that will be valued by anyone who owns it.

**Stephen J Ryan, MD**
President, Doheny Eye Institute
Professor, Department of Ophthalmology
Dean, University of Southern California School of Medicine
Los Angeles, California

# Introduction

The areas covered in this book are often thought of as tedious by many readers. This text covers specialized diagnostic tests, microbiology, psychophysical testing, ultrasonography and axial eye length measurements, electrophysiology, disability evaluation, and universal precautions. Many individuals will have little or no information on some of these subjects, while others will be quite familiar with some areas covered in this book. For some there is no personal desire to learn of these things, but it is knowledge that is required for certain levels of certification. However, I believe that after reading this book many of you will have a greater appreciation of the importance of some of the tests and techniques used in ophthalmology. This book is intended to be an introductory text designed to give you an overview of various specialized areas in the field of ophthalmology. Where appropriate, I have referred interested readers to other texts.

I have an extensive amount of clinical experience and have tried to bring that experience to this text. I use many case histories, some of which are taken directly from my lectures, whereas others are good examples of specific disease entities. Since this material can be difficult to get through, I have tried to keep the writing easy to understand and enjoyable. I used technical terms where appropriate, but tried not to get bogged down in excessive detail. I want the reader to learn enough to understand the test or procedure, but not so much as to go to sleep! My intent was not to create a substitute for sheep-counting, but rather a book that will impart the type of enthusiasm I have for these areas of ophthalmology.

The first section of the book is entitled Advanced Tests and Techniques. It includes a chapter on diagnostic tests which contains descriptions of such important and frequently used tests as pachymetry and corneal topography, as well as obsolete tests such as pupillography. The second chapter is on psychophysical testing. This chapter has brief descriptions of the macular stress, potential acuity, and glare tests. There is extensive writing on advanced color vision, dark adaptometry, and contrast sensitivity. (There are few books written for optometric and ophthalmic personnel that include such extensive treatment of these subjects.) The section concludes with a chapter on microbiology. This chapter discusses ocular microorganisms, identifying infectious agents, and a brief description of the human immune system.

The second section of the book is on biometry and echography. This section provides the reader with an overview of this very important aspect of the ophthalmic practice. It is designed to give you sufficient understanding of how and why the tests are performed. The third section of the book is on ocular electrophysiology. This is my favorite subject, and I hope my enthusiasm shows through! I have included extensive chapters on electroretinography, electro-oculography, and visual evoked response testing. Again, these tests are treated extensively in this book.

I have concluded this book with two important appendices. One is on disability determination and the other on universal precautions. The appendix on disability determination is designed as a "how to" chapter, and can be used as a reference when trying to determine if a particular patient qualifies for disability based on vision loss. The appendix on universal precautions was originally part of the microbiology chapter, as universal precautions help us eliminate the possibility of spreading ocular infections from one patient to another. My editor thought that it would better serve the readers if it were a separate appendix, and I have to agree with her. The reader should be able to use this appendix as a reference when questions of universal precaution guidelines within an eye practice are brought up.

Many hours of labor and love were put into this book. I certainly hope that you find it enjoyable reading, as well as helpful in your pursuit of knowledge in the field of eyecare.

# The Study Icons

*The Basic Bookshelf for Eyecare Professionals* is quality educational material designed for professionals in all branches of eyecare. Because so many of you want to expand your careers, we have made a special effort to include information needed for certification exams. When these study icons appear in the margin of a *Series* book, it is your cue that the material next to the icon (which may be a paragraph or an entire section) is listed as a criteria item for a certification examination. Please use this key to identify the appropriate icon:

**OptA**   optometric assistant

**OptT**   optometric technician

**OphA**   ophthalmic assistant

**OphT**   ophthalmic technician

**OphMT**   ophthalmic medical technologist*

**LV**   low vision subspecialty

**Srg**   ophthalmic surgical assisting subspecialty

**CL**   contact lens registry

**Optn**   opticianry

**RA**   retinal angiographer

*\*Because this icon applies to the entire text, (except where noted) it will not appear anywhere on the pages.*

Part I

# Advanced Tests and Techniques

Chapter 1

# Diagnostic Testing

**KEY POINTS**

- Diagnostic tests can be used to evaluate both the structure and function of the eye.

- Patients are not required to respond to an examiner when diagnostic tests are being performed.

- Many diagnostic tests are easy to perform and require minimal patient cooperation.

# Exophthalmometry

Exophthalmometry evaluates the forward protrusion of the eye by measuring the distance between the anterior surface of the cornea and the bony margin of the orbit. Forward protrusion can be bilateral (exophthalmos) or unilateral (proptosis), depending on the underlying cause. Protrusion of the eye can be caused by orbital tumors, trauma, inflammation, or disease; however, it is most commonly seen in patients who have thyroid disease. If ocular manifestations such as exophthalmos are present in the patient with thyroid disease, the patient is said to have Graves' disease. Since thyroid disease and tumors are normally progressive, it is critical to measure and monitor the degree of exophthalmos or proptosis at regular intervals.

Exophthalmos can be grossly viewed from above the patient; however, to accurately measure the degree of protrusion, one must use an instrument called an exophthalmometer. There are two types of exophthalmometers. The first (and oldest) type is the Leudde exophthalmometer. The Leudde is simply a clear plastic millimeter rule that is placed on the lateral bony orbit. The examiner stands to the patient's side at eye level, views the patient's cornea through the clear plastic rule, and notes the point at which the cornea aligns with the scale. The procedure is repeated on the other eye. The difference between the two eyes is then compared and recorded. A difference of 2 mm or more is considered indicative of proptosis. Because the Leudde exophthalmometer allows only a unilateral measurement and depends on subsequent examiners placing the instrument in the same exact spot, reliability is a concern.

The Hertel exophthalmometer allows for simultaneous measurement of the eyes. It also utilizes a calibrated base, allowing for more reliable repeatability of subsequent measurements. The Hertel consists of two measuring devices separated by a metal bar (Figure 1-1). The measuring devices each have two mirrors, so that a vertical profile of the patient's cornea and a measuring scale can be viewed simultaneously. The instrument may be used on all patients regardless of their size or facial symmetry. Because of its reliability, the Hertel is the preferred instrument.

To measure ocular protrusion with the Hertel, the examiner sits directly in front of the patient at eye level. The patient is instructed to look straight ahead (Figure 1-2). The outer edge of each measuring device has a small projection which is fit firmly on the lateral margin of both bony orbits. The right measuring device is moved until it fits firmly against the orbits. While the examiner is checking the patient's right eye, the patient is asked to fixate on the examiner's left eye. The examiner notes the reading where the cornea aligns on the scale. Without moving, the examiner views the patient's left eye with his or her own right eye. (The patient is asked to fixate on the examiner's right eye.) Again the examiner notes the reading on the scale. In addition, the base measurement (which is the distance between the two measuring devices) is noted, recorded, and used on all subsequent measurements to ensure continued accuracy.

The Hertel exophthalmometer provides reliable information about how far forward each eye is in comparison to both its bony orbit and the other eye. The normal range is between 12 and 20 mm. Readings over 20 mm suggest protrusion, and an underlying cause should be suspected. As with the Leudde exophthalmometer, a difference of two or more millimeters between the two eyes is considered significant.

# Pachymetry

Normal corneal thickness ranges from 1 mm at the very periphery of the cornea to 0.5 mm at the center. Some individuals have thinner or thicker corneas, and some corneal diseases result in

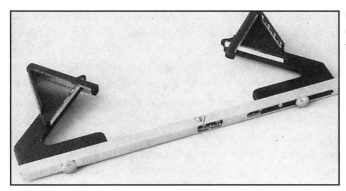

**Figure 1-1.** Exophthalmometer. (Photo courtesy of Leica Ophthalmic Instruments Division.)

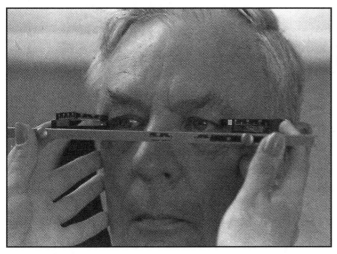

**Figure 1-2.** Performing exophthalmetry on a patient. (Photo by Mark Arrigoni. Reprinted with permission from Herrin MP. *Ophthalmic Examination and Basic Skills.* Thorofare, NJ: SLACK Incorporated; 1990.)

changes in corneal thickness (such as corneal thinning in keratoconus). The measurement of corneal thickness can be very useful in evaluating the integrity of the cornea, and is done with an instrument known as a pachymeter. There are two types of pachymeters; one is attached to the slit lamp, while the other is a free-standing ultrasonic device. The slit lamp version is used less frequently.

The slit lamp pachymeter can be used to measure either the depth of the anterior chamber or the thickness of the cornea. When the corneal thickness is being measured, a split beam is projected onto the cornea: one portion of the beam onto the corneal epithelium, the other onto the corneal endothelium. In order for the thickness of the cornea to be measured, the radius of the

## What the Patient Needs to Know

- This is a test to determine the thickness of your cornea.
- Your eye will be numbed with a local anesthetic that may sting a little.
- A small probe will touch the front of your eye. This will not hurt, but you will feel something touching your eye.
- Try to keep your eyes open during the test.
- It is important that you look at the fixation spot throughout the entire test. If you move your eyes excessively during this test, the results may not be accurate.

curvature of the cornea must also be obtained with the keratometer. This cumbersome means of testing corneal thickness requires mathematical calculations, and has been replaced by the ultrasonic pachymeter (which is also easier to use).

The ultrasonic pachymeter is small and portable, thus allowing its use without the need of a slit lamp. A probe, somewhat similar to that of an A-scan probe, is placed directly on the cornea. Sound waves pass through the cornea, yielding a measurement of its thickness. The measurements are seen on the pachymeter display and are given in microns.

A straight probe tip is used to measure the central cornea and an angled tip is used for the periphery (Figure 1-3). Accurate corneal thickness can only be obtained if the probe is perpendicular to the cornea. This is easy to do in the central corneal area, as the anterior and posterior surfaces of the cornea are the most parallel at this point. More peripheral areas of the cornea are not as parallel, thus making it especially difficult to put the pachymetry probe perpendicular to the test area. This is particularly problematic when the extreme peripheral areas of the cornea are being measured. If the probe is not perpendicular with the cornea, the reading will register thicker than the tissue actually is. Care must be taken to ensure that the measurements are as accurate as possible, because such information may be used for surgical calculations. Accuracy in corneal measuring can be enhanced by good testing techniques.

## Performing Pachymetry

It is important to make the patient as comfortable as possible for this exam (Figure 1-4). A reclining chair is ideal, but not always feasible. A clinic examination room or room where ultrasonography is performed would also be appropriate.

The patient is told that a probe will be touching the front of the eye, but that there will be no pain involved. The patient should be encouraged not to move his or her eye, and should be told not to blink or squeeze the eyelids.

First the eye is anesthetized with a local anesthetic. The patient is then asked to look straight ahead at the fixation target. The technician should start by measuring the center-most portion of the cornea (Figure 1-5). The straight probe is placed perpendicularly on the center of the cornea. Several readings should be taken and the different thicknesses should be averaged for the final reading.

Mapping the thickness of the peripheral cornea with the angled probe can be accomplished by one of two techniques (Figure 1-6). One technique is to follow imaginary concentric rings around the center of the cornea. The center is measured first, then the probe is moved away from the center by about 1 mm, and a 3 mm diameter ring is measured. After that ring is successfully measured, the probe is moved out an additional millimeter and a second ring of about a 7 mm diameter is measured. The second method is to measure the central area first (as previously described), then move the probe out along a similar radius from the center to the periphery. Do this along eight radii of the eye until the entire thickness of the entire cornea has been mapped. Care must be taken to keep the probe perpendicular to the anterior cornea. The machine might not register a numeric value if the probe is sufficiently misaligned (Figure 1-7). Always start with the central cornea, as this is the thinnest area in the normal cornea. This numeric value can be used to support peripheral corneal thickness values.

One disadvantage of most ultrasonic pachymeters is that they do not provide the actual echogram, as would be the case in axial eye length or diagnostic A- and B-scan ultrasonography. Therefore, the technician must rely on how the probe looks on the patient's eye as well as the appropriateness of the numeric value displayed on the screen.

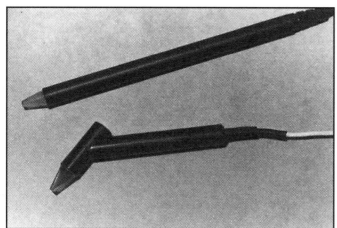

**Figure 1-3.** Two different pachymetry probes, straight and angled tips. (Reprinted with permission from Kendall CJ. *Ophthalmic Echography*. Thorofare, NJ: SLACK Incorporated; 1990.)

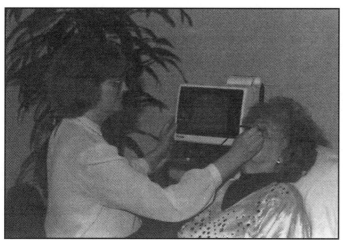

**Figure 1-4.** Positioning of the patient's head near the instrument is an important part of good technique. (Reprinted with permission from Kendall CJ. *Ophthalmic Echography*. Thorofare, NJ: SLACK Incorporated; 1990.)

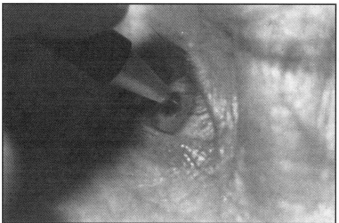

**Figure 1-5.** Central corneal thickness is being measured. Note the angle of the probe is perpendicular to both corneal surfaces. (Reprinted with permission from Kendall CJ. *Ophthalmic Echography*. Thorofare, NJ: SLACK Incorporated; 1990.)

**Figure 1-6.** Peripheral corneal measurement being made. Note the different probe angle from the central reading. The sound beam is perpendicular to the peripheral corneal surfaces. (Reprinted with permission from Kendall CJ. *Ophthalmic Echography*. Thorofare, NJ: SLACK Incorporated; 1990.)

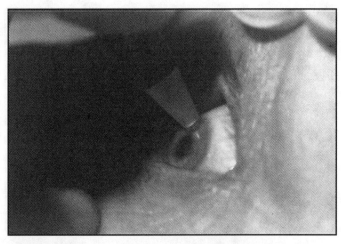

**Figure 1-7.** Off-axis peripheral corneal scan probably produces no measurements or a falsely thick one. The probe is not perpendicular to the corneal surfaces. (Reprinted with permission from Kendall CJ. *Ophthalmic Echography*. Thorofare, NJ: SLACK Incorporated; 1990.)

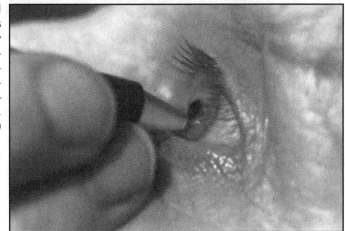

# Photokeratoscopy

The photokeratoscope is a device used to evaluate the anterior surface of the cornea. It is a photographic unit with a cone-shaped section containing a series of concentric rings similar to that of the Placido's disk (Figure 1-8). An eyepiece on the other end allows the technician to view the patient's eye. The rings are illuminated and projected onto the cornea at the same time as a picture is taken. The resulting photograph provides a graphic representation of the anterior corneal surface (Figure 1-9).

## Performing Photokeratoscopy

The patient sits with his or her head securely on a chin rest. The instrument can be moved so that the technician can project the image onto either eye. Prior to taking the photograph, the patient should close his or her eyes to make sure that the surface of the cornea is moist. (A dry cornea can appear to be irregularly shaped, but this irregularity should not wind up in a patient's chart.)

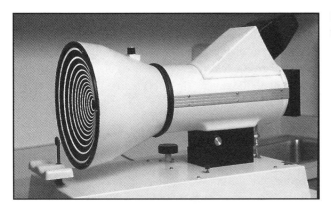

**Figure 1-8.** Photokeratoscope. (Photograph by Nilo Davila.)

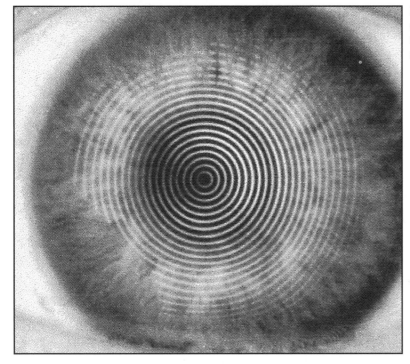

**Figure 1-9.** An image of a normal cornea using a photokeratoscope.

The technician adjusts the image of the rings with a focusing knob. It is important that the central portion of the cornea is properly aligned and the rings in this area are in focus prior to the picture being taken, because poor alignment and focus may result in erroneous findings. If the central portion is properly in focus, the eye is adequately moist, and the patient's head is properly aligned, then other areas of the cornea that are not in focus represent true irregularities. Such irregularities may have clinical or diagnostic significance. The patient is asked to keep the eye wide open during the actual photograph. Care should be taken to ensure that the eye is fully opened, as the lids can interfere with a good photograph.

This test is useful in evaluating the presence of corneal irregularities such as post-operative astigmatism, severe corneal flattening after grafting, or the presence of an extremely steep cornea as in keratoconus. This information might be used by the physician to justify contact lens fitting or corrective refractive surgery.

In eyes with flat corneas, the rings will be spaced farther apart than normal. Steep corneas will have rings that are spaced closer together than normal. In individuals with astigmatism, the rings on one axis will be spaced similarly, while the rings on the perpendicular axis will be spaced significantly differently (either closer or farther apart). In eyes with corneal irregularities due to disease, scarring, or corneal surgery, the rings will be irregularly shaped (Figures 1-10 and 1-11).

**CL**

# Corneal Topography*

Corneal topography creates a computerized map of the surface of the cornea. This map is an essential part of all preoperative evaluations for refractive surgery. The map of the cornea is similar to any topographic map in which steep areas are represented by one color and shallow areas by another color. In corneal topography, the steep portions of the cornea are represented by dark red and red (keratometry [K] readings in the high 40s or low 50s), whereas the shallow areas are represented in blue and purple (K readings in the mid 30s). Corneas that are in the medium range of steepness are represented by green (K readings in the mid 40s).

The topographic colors are not absolutely fixed to specific K readings, but represent the relative relationship of steepness and flatness of the cornea. The legend must always be used to determine the specific K readings for any particular color.

A spherically shaped cornea of moderate steepness would appear almost completely green on a topographic map. Corneas with significant astigmatism will produce a typical hourglass shape in one color along one axis, and along the opposite axis another color will appear. One axis might appear red and the other yellow (or in flatter corneas, yellow and green), thus suggesting that one axis is steeper than the other. In irregularly shaped corneas, this hourglass pattern will not appear. Instead, one area of the cornea will be steep, but the area across from it may not be as steep. This pattern is more likely to appear in patients who have undergone penetrating keratoplasty, have some type of corneal problem (such as keratoconus), or who have had a cataract extraction. These irregular patterns are generally not seen in patients with healthy corneas.

## Performing Corneal Topography

The patient is seated in front of the unit, and asked to look straight ahead (Figure 1-12). When the patient's right eye is being tested, his or her head is turned slightly to the left. This eliminates any potential artifacts from the face (shadows). The patient is asked to blink periodically to ensure that the cornea is moist, which results in sharper images.

The patient is asked to look straight ahead at a fixation target. On a computer screen adjacent to the topography unit, the examiner sees the patient's eye with rings projected onto it (similar to those seen in the photokeratoscope) (Figure 1-13). Once the examiner has a clear and focused view of the ring-covered cornea, the image is captured by pressing a button on a joystick or clicking on a mouse, depending on the unit. The image is then analyzed by the computer. If the computer determines that the image is reliable, it will then "draw" a series of colored rings on top of the corneal image from the center of the cornea to the mid-periphery. If the computer does not think that the image is reliable, then the colored image will not appear, signaling the examiner to "try again." Once the examiner has obtained an image that the computer has analyzed as reliable, a second screen appears. This gives the exact level of reliability of the image as analyzed by the computer. Reliability is presented as a confidence level, from high to low, based on such things as focus and centering of the cornea. If the examiner finds

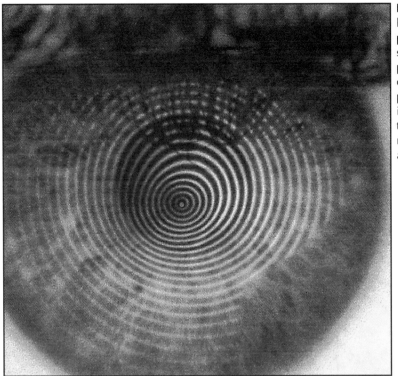

**Figure 1-10.** Irregularly shaped corneas produce irregularly shaped rings. This patient has keratoconus. The lower portion of the cornea is steeper as noted by the narrowing of the rings on the inferior aspect of the cornea.

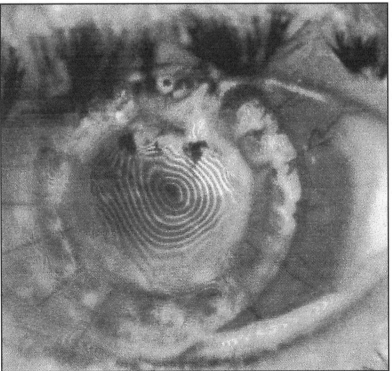

**Figure 1-11.** An image of a patient who has undergone penetrating keratoplasty. Note the sutures in the peripheral cornea. There is significant astigmatism as noted by the irregularity of the mires.

**Figure 1-12.** Patient properly seated at a corneal topography unit. (Photograph by Nilo Davila.)

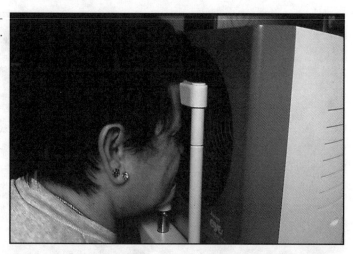

**Figure 1-13.** Image of the cornea seen by the technician performing corneal topography. (Photograph by Nilo Davila.)

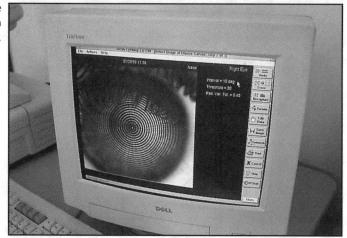

the level of reliability to be acceptable, the image is saved for later use. Patient demographics (such as age, sex, and eye) are saved as well.

The examiner can print the image on a color printer immediately after the test has been completed. The printed chart looks nothing like that seen on the screen. In fact, if someone did not know that he or she was looking at a topographic map of the eye, there would be no clues present to indicate that fact. The image looks very similar to a round island (Figure 1-14). The patient's demographic information appears on the side of the image with a legend, so that the topographic map can be read for curvature. The computer does not draw rings, but fills in the non-tested spaces by extrapolating data based on the relationship of adjacent rings. If the computer did not do this, then the printout would look similar to the image produced by the photokeratoscope.

The mathematical formula in the computer's program creates a topographic representation of the entire cornea. This information can be used by the ophthalmologist prior to refractive surgery. Additionally, the topographic image of the cornea can be used to more accurately analyze corneal curvature in diseased corneas, or in residual postoperative astigmatism.

*The information in this section does not appear on the ophthalmic technology exam.*

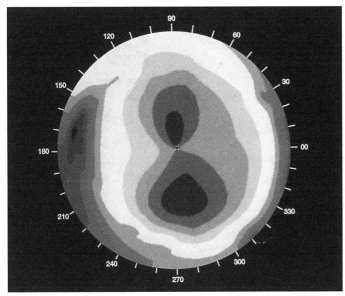

**Figure 1-14.** Topographic image of the cornea. This image is produced in color with a legend printed on the side to illustrate which colors correspond to specific K readings. Dark reds are associated with steeper corneas. Astigmatic corneas will produce this appearance where colors along the same axis will be similar; the colors of opposing axes will be different.

## What the Patient Needs to Know

- This is a test to evaluate the curvature of the front of your eye.
- A map will be drawn of the front of your eye based on its shape; this map will look similar to other topographic maps that you have seen.
- This map will be used by your doctor to evaluate your cornea.
- Place your chin on the chin rest, keep your eyes wide open, and try not to move around.
- It is important that you watch the fixation device closely.
- Try not to blink excessively, but do blink fully when told to close your eye.

# Pupillometry*

During the examination of the pupils, the patient should face a light source so the general size, shape, and symmetry of the pupils can be noted. Although these are very important features of pupillary evaluation, there is one significant drawback. They require subjective estimations by the examiner. A means by which to reduce subjectivity has been the goal of many eyecare providers.

An easy means by which to evaluate the size of a pupil is to compare it to circular disks of graduating (and known) sizes. These disks are frequently printed on near vision cards (Figure 1-15). The pupillometer is a more sophisticated device for measuring pupil size, although it is rarely used. The pupillometer is held in front of the patient's eye at a specified distance. The examiner views the patient's pupil through the device. A numeric scale is projected onto the pupil, providing an accurate pupil size. This is a static measurement.

*The information in this section does not appear on the ophthalmic technology exam.*

**Figure 1-15.** Near vision card with a series of graduated semicircles (bottom) to be used to estimate pupillary diameter. (Photograph by Nilo Davila.)

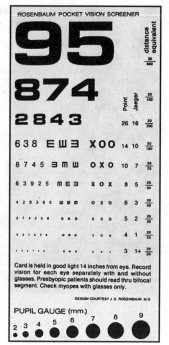

# Pupillography

The pupil is a dynamic sphincter muscle, and its actions can reveal significant ocular pathologies or anomalies. The need for dynamic evaluation of the pupil resulted in the photographic and cinematographic testing of pupillary responses. The purpose of pupillography is to obtain an accurate photographic representation of the undilated pupil. Regular photography with standard illumination results in a constricted pupil in many instances, unless the exposure time is so short that the photograph is taken before the pupil can react to the flash. To eliminate this potential problem, and to obtain photographic records of the dark-adapted pupil, infrared lighting is used during pupillography. When using infrared light, the pupil does not respond to the photographic light source, but only the ambient lighting. Additionally, in an eye with a mild corneal opacity, the infrared light can penetrate the opacity and reveal the shadow of the pupil through the opacification. Both static and dynamic responses of the pupil can be observed via this method.

Although pupillography using infrared lighting provides a direct representation of the unstimulated pupil, the dynamic aspects of pupillary functioning are not adequately captured by this method. Cinematographic (motion picture) documentation of pupillary responses achieves this goal. While using an infrared light source, a video of pupillary responses to various conditions is recorded. Both eyes are recorded simultaneously, but the edited version consists of only the two eyes without any other features so that the pupillary response can be measured. A graph is created that represents pupil size over time. The direct pupillary reaction and the consensual pupillary action are recorded separately. The width of the pupils decreases as one pupil is exposed to a white light, and then increases in size when the light stimulus is eliminated. The graph shows how quickly each pupil reacts to light. Time is measured in seconds.

Although pupillometry and pupillography seem like useful diagnostic tools, they have not been used widely for many years. Most of the research on these devices was conducted at the end of the 19th century and the beginning of the 20th century.

# Ophthalmoscopy

## Introduction

Ophthalmoscopy is very much like looking into a round room through a tiny, round window. As you can imagine, it would be very hard to see the entire room. Ophthalmoscopy is the examination of the internal structures of the posterior chamber of the eye through the tiny window of the pupil.

While an eye examination is not a substitute for a complete physical examination, many systemic diseases that exhibit ocular manifestations have been diagnosed simply by the appearance of the retinal vasculature of the eye. Disorders such as diabetes mellitus, high blood pressure, vascular disorders, blood disorders, intracranial tumors, and certain other systemic diseases can cause ocular manifestations that are easily seen and monitored with the ophthalmoscope. Ophthalmoscopy is an integral part of the diagnosis and management of ocular diseases such as glaucoma, ocular lesions, abnormalities, and trauma (including retinal detachment).

## Dilation

Since most pupils are large enough to afford a satisfactory examination of the optic nerve head and the surrounding retinal areas, direct ophthalmoscopy can be performed through an undilated pupil; however, dilation of the pupil is necessary for a thorough ophthalmoscopic examination utilizing either the direct or the indirect ophthalmoscope. Dilation should be achieved by using a cycloplegic agent which will not only dilate the pupil but will also paralyze the ciliary body, thereby paralyzing accommodation and ensuring that the pupil will remain dilated when the bright examination light is used. Mydriasis alone will not allow the pupil to remain widely dilated in the presence of a bright direct light. A short-acting cycloplegic such as tropicamide 0.5 to 1% along with the mydriatic, phenylephrine hydrochloride 2.5%, will produce adequate dilation in 15 to 20 minutes and will wear off in 2 to 4 hours.

Of course, dilation should not be performed until the appropriate pupillary examinations have been performed. The presence of abnormal pupillary reactions, inequality of pupil size, abnormal speed of response to light and/or accommodation indicate that a non-dilated ophthalmoscopic examination should be performed first.

In addition, dilation should be performed only after careful assessment of the anterior chamber angle. The angle can be easily evaluated by placing a light source at the temporal side of the patient's eye near the cornea. If there is an apparent space between the cornea and the angle, then the angle is likely deep. If there is a shadow at the nasal side of the angle, or the iris looks as if it is against the cornea, then the angle is likely narrow. (This can be better evaluated with a slit lamp beam, but the principle is the same.) If the angle is narrow, then it may be advisable to check with the physician prior to dilating the patient, as individuals with narrow angles can be at risk for attacks of angle-closure glaucoma. Angle-closure glaucoma occurs when the pupil is dilated and the excess iris fills in the angle, thus closing off the outflow mechanism of the eye. Aqueous backs up, causing an extreme spike in intraocular pressure (IOP), with associated pain and redness in the eye. Patients frequently complain of nausea as well. Narrow angle glaucoma accounts for only a small number of glaucoma cases, and is usually seen in middle-aged hyperopic patients.

## Instrumentation

Two types of ophthalmoscopes may be utilized in performing the ophthalmoscopic examination. The direct ophthalmoscope and the indirect ophthalmoscope each have distinct advantages and disadvantages (Table 1-1).

### Direct Ophthalmoscopy

Direct ophthalmoscopy can be performed through an undilated pupil; however, the view is limited to the fundus area (disk and macula). It requires only the use of a direct ophthalmoscope. The direct ophthalmoscope is a hand-held instrument which can be powered by battery or electricity, and is more convenient if portability is desired (Figures 1-16 and 1-17).

Since most patients are not emmetropic (without refractive error), the direct ophthalmoscope's head contains a wheel of plus and minus spheres for the neutralization of myopia (minus spheres) or hyperopia (plus spheres). The minus lenses are designated by red numbers and the plus by black. Dialing in these lenses will bring the posterior pole into sharp view (Figure 1-18).

Most direct ophthalmoscopes have two round apertures intended for use with small and large pupils respectively, a slit, a grid, and a green (or red-free) filter (Figure 1-19). The slit is used to determine the elevation or depression of retinal lesions. When using the slit, it is important that the examiner view the lesion by allowing the slit to fall both on the lesion as well as surrounding normal retina. A flat lesion will not distort the vertical slit, but an elevated lesion will cause a bowing of the slit with the convexity of the beam closest to the examiner. A depression will cause a bowing of the slit away from the examiner, with the undistorted sections of the beam appearing closest to the examiner.

Since the direct ophthalmoscope is a monocular instrument and provides a monocular view, depth perception is not present. Without the use of the slit beam, elevations and depressions would be very difficult to gauge.

The grid is used as a measuring device. When the grid is projected over a vessel or lesion, the number of spaces in the grid filled by the vessel or lesion is counted and recorded for future comparison.

The green filter provides a red-free light that is very useful in detecting small aneurysms and hemorrhages that might go unnoticed with standard light, but stand out nicely with the use of the green filter. (Blood and blood vessels appear black with red-free light.) The red-free light is also useful in viewing the retinal nerve fibers.

The view through the direct ophthalmoscope is upright. Magnification through the direct ophthalmoscope is approximately 14 times the actual object size; however, the field of view is limited to only approximately 10 degrees. With direct ophthalmoscopy, only structures posterior to the equator can be seen and evaluated.

When evaluating the patient's right eye, hold the instrument in your right hand and use your own right eye. The patient's left eye is viewed with your left eye, holding the instrument in your left hand. Dim the lights and ask the patient to look straight ahead at a specified target. Start with the focus wheel on a higher plus lens and center the light on the patient's pupil, beginning at about 24 inches away. Steadily move closer to the patient, keeping the light centered on the pupil. You will first see the cornea, then the iris, then the lens. Begin dialing the focus wheel toward the

Table 1-1.
## Comparison of Direct and Indirect Ophthalmoscopy

| **Direct** | **Indirect** |
|---|---|
| Dilated or undilated pupil | Widely dilated pupil |
| Monocular view | Binocular stereoscopic view |
| Small field of view (approx. 10 degrees) | Larger 45 degree field of view |
| Approximately 14x magnification | 2x to 4x depending on lens used |
| Upright, non-reversed view | Inverted and reversed view |
| Hand-held | Worn on the head of the examiner |
| No condensing lens necessary | Hand-held condensing lens necessary |

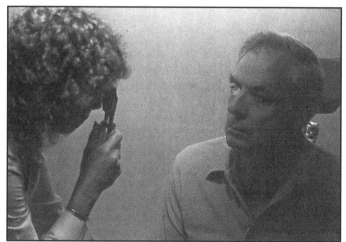

**Figure 1-16.** The right eye is used to examine the patient's right eye and the left eye is used to examine the left eye. (Photo by Mark Arrigoni. Reprinted with permission from Herrin MP. *Ophthalmic Examination and Basic Skills.* Thorofare, NJ: SLACK Incorporated; 1990.)

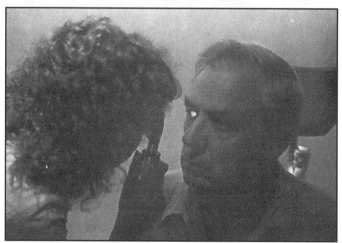

**Figure 1-17.** Keep the light focused on the eye while moving closer toward the patient. (Photo by Mark Arrigoni. Reprinted with permission from Herrin MP. *Ophthalmic Examination and Basic Skills.* Thorofare, NJ: SLACK Incorporated; 1990.)

**Figure 1-18.** Rotate the lenses to neutralize any refractive error that may exist. (Photo by Mark Arrigoni. Reprinted with permission from Herrin MP. *Ophthalmic Examination and Basic Skills.* Thorofare, NJ: SLACK Incorporated; 1990.)

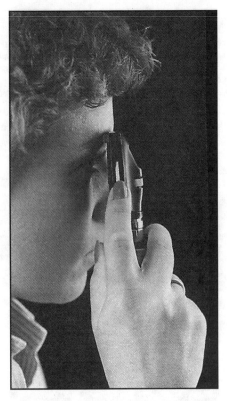

**Figure 1-19.** Filters are changed by rotating the white ring. (Photo by Mark Arrigoni. Reprinted with permission from Herrin MP. *Ophthalmic Examination and Basic Skills.* Thorofare, NJ: SLACK Incorporated; 1990.)

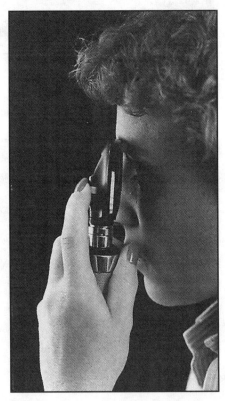

minus as you move in closer. For the retinal examination, you will be only 1 to 2 inches from the patient's eye. To help control your own accommodation, try to focus your vision far away, as if you are looking *through* the patient's eye. You may need to brace the hand holding the ophthalmoscope against the patient's cheek to help steady your hand.

Once the retina is in focus, find the optic nerve. This is easily done by following any retinal vessel to the disk. The disk is evaluated for shape, size, and color. Just temporal to the disk (about two disk diameters) is the macula, at the center of which is the fovea. After examining the macula, follow each of the major retinal vessels outward from the disk as far as you can. You may need to turn the instrument horizontally to view the 12:00 to 6:00 positions.

## Indirect Ophthalmoscopy

The indirect ophthalmoscope is a binocular instrument that is worn on the head of the examiner. An aspheric condensing lens (loupe) is held at approximately arm's length and is manipulated to bring the fundus into sharp view (Figure 1-20). The image the examiner observes is inverted and reversed. Because the instrument is binocular, a stereoscopic view of the entire fundus is possible. This view is very useful in identifying and assessing elevations and depressions in the ocular fundus. Depending on the power of the hand-held condensing lens used, the indirect ophthalmoscope affords only a 2x to 4x magnification of actual size; however, structures anterior to the equator, as far as the ora serrata, may be observed and evaluated by indenting the sclera with a scleral depressor (Figure 1-21). Indirect ophthalmoscopy must be performed through a widely dilated pupil.

Indirect ophthalmoscopy is best performed with the patient lying down. This way you are free to move about the patient's head to obtain the best view. The condensing lens can be held with your thumb and forefinger, freeing your other fingers to help hold the patient's lower lid down. The upper lid can be held with your free hand. The condensing lens is positioned several inches from the patient's eye and focused on the retinal area of interest. The light should be focused on the retina for only a few seconds at a time, then moved aside briefly. The patient is directed to look into various gazes to allow you to view all areas of the retina. (Simply ask the patient to look toward the quadrant that you wish to examine.) Remember, however, that the image you are seeing is inverted and reversed.

If you have trouble focusing the retina, try moving a bit closer to or farther away from the patient. If lens reflections are bothersome, try tilting the lens just a little. This maneuver is especially useful when viewing the periphery, because oblique astigmatism comes into play due to the angle (through the patient's media) which you are looking.

**Figure 1-20.** Examiner with an indirect ophthalmoscope and condensing lens. The image that is seen is reversed, but two-dimensional. (Photograph by Nilo Davila.)

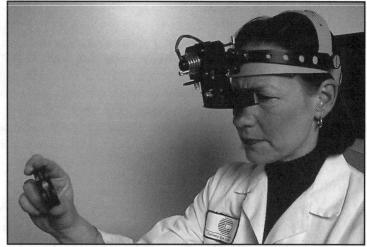

**Figure 1-21.** Scleral depressor. This is held in the examiner's hand and is used to depress the sclera while observing the area of the ora serrata with the indirect ophthalmoscope. (Photograph by Nilo Davila.)

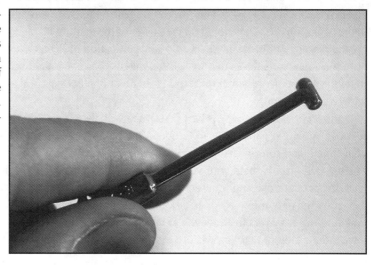

# Psychophysical Testing

- Psychophysical tests provide information about how an individual perceives his or her world.

- The tests require direct patient input, and can be influenced by such things as patient cooperation level, understanding, and age.

- Psychophysical test results may not be reliable, because patient factors influence the results.

# Overview of Psychophysical Testing

Psychophysical tests are conducted to determine how an individual perceives his or her world. These tests require subjective responses that can be influenced by such things as the patient's cooperation and age. The most common psychophysical test conducted by ancillary personnel in the eyecare setting is visual acuity testing. We are asking the patient to tell us how well he or she can differentiate high contrast items at varying distances. A toddler cannot tell us because a child that young does not understand what we are asking of him or her. An uncooperative patient might report that he or she cannot see any of the letters when, in fact, the person has no real visual problems. Therefore, psychophysical testing is not appropriate for all individuals, and can produce misleading results in those who are not being accurate. In these instances objective tests such as the ERG, EOG, and VER can provide more accurate estimations of how a person sees. However, such diagnostic tests do not reveal the subtleties of vision. The best way to know how a person sees is to ask the individual directly. This chapter will be dedicated to describing the usefulness of such subjective tests, including color vision, dark adaptation, contrast sensitivity, and glare. Remember, all of the tests in this section require the patient to tell us how he or she sees. The patient's response is then compared against preestablished normative values.

# Advanced Color Vision Testing

## Mechanisms of Normal Color Vision

The cone photoreceptors allow the perception of color. In order for a person to see color normally, the individual must have properly functioning cones, each with one of three visual pigments. These visual pigments determine which wavelength of light a particular cone will be most sensitive to. The cones are either most sensitive to reddish light, greenish light, or bluish light. Normal color vision is therefore trichromatic, and normal color vision depends on the relative activity of all three cone types. For example, if a wavelength of light entering the eye stimulates both red cones and blue cones, the person perceives that the object is purple. This relative activity of the three cone types provides the normal observer with over 200 different color sensations.

## Color Vision Abnormalities

Although we might want to spend time evaluating individuals with normal color vision, our main concern as ancillary staff is to identify and evaluate those individuals with color vision deficiencies. Color vision defects can be classified as either congenital or acquired. Once that differentiation has been made, we can determine if the defect is mild, moderate, severe, or absolute. Finally, we can identify which specific color mechanism is involved.

### Onset

Congenital color vision defects are those present at birth. The inheritance pattern is generally X-linked recessive, where the carrier mother gives the defective gene to her son who manifests the symptoms. Since the defect is present from birth, there is no ongoing change in the patient's color perception. The patient will produce similar test findings, suggesting one type of color mechanism, regardless of the type of color vision test being employed. Furthermore, the patient can undergo the same test over a 10 year period and the results will be virtually identical every time. This is due to the stable nature of the congenital color vision defect. Generally, there are no other ocular problems and the individual has normal vision in all other respects.

Acquired color vision defects, on the other hand, occur over time. A person could be born with normal color vision, but because of some type of abnormality (such as glaucoma or drug sensitivity), will start to lose his or her color perception. When examined using different types of color vision tests this person will produce different types of results. The individual might make mistakes on one test that suggest that the green pigment is involved, while on a second test the results might implicate the blue pigment. Moreover, if the patient was tested over a 10-year period the color vision results would change, more than likely getting worse as time goes on. Some individuals with severe problems develop achromatopsia (they see in black and white). This can occur in individuals with cone dystrophy. Generally their photopic ERG is non-recordable (see Chapter 6).

Acquired color vision defects are almost always associated with other ocular abnormalities, such as retinal or optic nerve disease. Frequently these patients have reduced visual acuity, and sometimes the two eyes are not equally involved. Therefore, a patient may have significant abnormality in one eye with severe color vision deficiency, while the other eye is very nearly normal. Each eye may have color vision abnormalities that represent different color mechanisms as well.

## Severity

In the person with an acquired defect, level of severity will change over time and variability of severity may be noted between the two eyes. Those with congenital color vision defects show no variability over time, and severity is generally easier to establish.

Color vision defects can be either mild, moderate, severe (also known as incomplete color deficiencies), or complete. Those with mild, moderate, or severe color vision defects are considered to be *anomalous trichromats* as all three cone pigments are present, but one of the pigments is insufficient. (Normal trichromatic color vision is based on the presence of "equal" pigment from all three cone types.) The individual will be able to see some shades of the affected color, but not all. For instance, there may be a defect of the red mechanism. If the defect is mild, the individual might not be able to tell subtle differences in red hues. The person with a moderate defect might be able to see only very bright or saturated red colors, and might confuse certain red hues with certain green hues. The person with a severe defect will confuse almost all hues of red and green.

The person with a complete color vision defect has at least one of the cone pigments missing from the retina. One type of complete color vision defect results in the complete absence of only one color mechanism. This individual is considered a *dichromat*. (Dichromatic color vision means that only two cone pigment types are present.) The absent pigment is usually red or green, and the individual confuses all red shades with all green shades.

Another type of complete color defect involves two color mechanisms, where only one cone pigment type is present. This complete defect is refered to as monochromatism, where only one cone pigment is present. The *monochromat* is missing both the red and green pigments, while the blue pigment remains. This is known as blue cone monochromatism. This is an extremely rare color vision defect, and not one generally seen in a typical eye clinic. These individuals have severely abnormal color vision, reduced visual acuity, and abnormal cone ERGs (see Chapter 6).

A third complete color vision defect involves all three color mechanisms, where only rods are present in the eye. This individual has *achromatopsia*, which means a complete absence of color vision. (This defect is also referred to as rod monochromatism.) This individual sees in black, white, and shades of gray only. This is a fairly rare color vision defect, but one that may be seen several times per year in a university setting. These individuals have a complete absence of color vision, reduced visual acuity, and non-recordable cone ERGs (see Chapter 6). An incomplete *achromatopsia* can also occur. These individuals are very difficult to distinguish from those with blue cone monochromatism.

### Color Mechanism

Abnormality of the red color mechanism is referred to as a protan color defect. This causes confusion between red and green colors. Protan inheritance is X-linked recessive, with a 1% incidence rate for both complete (dichromat) and incomplete (anomalous trichromat) varieties (Table 2-1).

Abnormality of the green color mechanism is referred to as a deutan color defect. This causes confusion between red and green colors. Protan and deutan defects are often linked together by the expression "red/green color defect." This is not correct. It is more accurate to state the actual defect, such as a deutan defect. Both the protan and the deutan defects result in red/green confusion; however, those individuals with a complete protan defect have a worse color vision deficiency, as these individuals do not see any of the colors in the red spectrum. Therefore the actual visual spectrum that is seen by an individual with a complete protan defect is reduced. Those with a deutan defect can see the entire visible spectrum; however, these individuals do not see it correctly. As a result, knowing which type of defect is present helps determine the extent of the color vision loss. Deutan inheritance is also X-linked recessive. A complete dichromatic deutan defect occurs in 1% of the population, while the anomalous trichromatic defect occurs in about 5% of the population (see Table 2-1).

Abnormality of the blue color mechanism is referred to as a tritan color defect. This defect causes the individual to confuse blue and yellow colors. Tritan defects are very rare and are usually acquired rather than congenital. They are frequently associated with optic nerve diseases such as glaucoma or optic neuritis. The blue color mechanism seems particularly sensitive to the toxic effects of drugs and other pathologic conditions. A tritan defect that is congenital will result in a stationary color vision abnormality, whereas an acquired tritan defect will result in variability of color vision over time (see Table 2-1).

## Advanced Color Vision Tests

There are several types of advanced color vision tests that are commercially available and can be used to detect subtle color vision defects or to quantify the severity of the defect. The types of tests to be reviewed are the arrangement tests and matching tests (anomaloscope). Color vision plates are described in the Basic Bookshelf series book *Basic Procedures*.

### Arrangement Tests

Several types of arrangement tests are commercially available. The common principle of all arrangement tests is that they mimic a color wheel. The patient is asked to arrange the colored caps into a graded color order that should look somewhat like a rainbow. The correct arrangement of caps reveals the patient's ability to see subtle color gradation. If the patient has abnormal color vision, then the cap arrangement will reveal the type of color vision mechanism that is involved (a protan, deutan, or tritan defect). If the arrangement is abnormal, it is because the patient is confusing two very distinct colors that are opposite on the color wheel.

Table 2-1.
# Congenital Color Vision Defects (Nonprogressive) Categorized by Findings

| NAME | INHERITANCE | PRINCIPAL FINDINGS |
|---|---|---|
| **Group: Anomalous Trichromatism** | | In this group, patients match colors with all three primary pigments but use different proportions of each to make matches. Patients are usually asymptomatic with normal vision, and the diagnosis is made by color testing with an anomaloscope. |
| Protanomaly (1%) | X-L | Red deficiency |
| Deuteranomaly (5%) | X-L | Green deficiency |
| Tritanomaly (very rare) | | Blue deficiency |
| **Group: Dichromatism** | | In this group, patients match colors using only two colors. Visual acuity is normal, and the patients manifest "color confusion." This group includes the common red green color blindness. |
| Protanopia (1%) | X-L | Red mechanism absent (red green confusion) |
| Deuteranopia (1%) | X-L | Green mechanism absent (red green confusion) |
| Tritanopia (0.005%) | AD | Blue mechanism absent (blue yellow confusion) |
| **Group: Monochromatism** | | |
| Rod monochromatism (achromatism) | AR | Complete type: visual acuity is 20/200 Incomplete type: visual acuity is 20/40 to 20/100 Complete: virtual absence of color vision (Sloan test) Incomplete: abnormal color vision Photophobia, nystagmus, usually normal fundus with decreased foveal reflex; ERG photopic abnormal, ERG scotopic normal; photophobia and nystagmus may be minimal in the incomplete type, or may diminish after the second decade |
| Cone monochromatism (atypical monochromatism) | Unknown | Visual acuity is 20/20 Severely abnormal color vision, no photophobia, no nystagmus, fundus normal, postreceptor abnormality showing a normal photopic and scotopic ERG |
| Central cone monochromatism | AR | Visual acuity is 20/200 Only the macular cones are affected: photophobia, nystagmus; color vision mildly affected; normal photopic and scotopic ERG; close to normal flicker frequency |
| Blue cone monochromatism (atypical incomplete rod monochromatism) | X-L | Visual acuity is 20/60 to 20/200 No photophobia, minimal nystagmus, blue cones are minimally involved or not at all; abnormal photopic ERG, normal scotopic ERG; female carriers may show psychophysical and electrophysiologic abnormalities |

*Reprinted with permission from Jimenez-Sierra JM, Ogden TE, Van Boemel GB.* Inherited Retinal Diseases: A Diagnostic Guide. *St. Louis, Mo: CV Mosby Co.; 1989.*

The test requires that the patient has sufficient vision to see the caps, as well as sufficient cognitive skills in order to perform the test. The tests are not suitable for very young children or any others who may not be cooperative. The tests are qualitative in nature and reveal only the type of color mechanism involved, not its severity.

### Administering an Arrangement Test

All of the arrangement tests should be conducted in a similar manner. It is important that each eye be tested separately. This is very important when trying to determine if the defect is acquired, because acquired defects may produce different color abnormalities in each eye. The patient should be tested with his or her best spectacle correction, and undilated. Finally, the test should be conducted with a recommended light source such as the Sol Source Daylight Desk Lamp (Munsell Division of GreytagMacBeth, New Windsor, NY) that mimics sunlight. If it is not possible to use a standard light, use the same lighting condition with every patient and test several dozen normal patients to determine the upper limits of normal for the test under this lighting condition.

The examiner should mix up the colored caps (either on the desk or in the box) and then tell the patient to rearrange to caps in a graded color order. Remind the patient not to touch the colored portion of the caps, as oils from the fingers can discolor the caps. (If the caps become discolored they must be replaced. Replacement caps can be ordered from the companies that make the tests.)

**Figure 2-1.** Farnsworth-Munsell D-15 Panel and Sol Source Daylight Desk Lamp. (Photograph by Ronald Morales.)

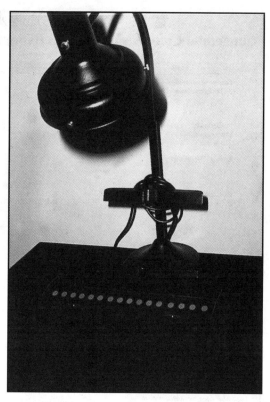

## What the Patient Needs to Know

- This is a test to evaluate your color vision.
- Arrange the caps in color order so they form a series from one end to the other.
- Your color vision will be tested one eye at a time.
- Please do not touch the colored part of the caps.

### Farnsworth-Munsell D-15 Panel

The Farnsworth-Munsell D-15 Panel (Munsell Division of GreytagMacBeth, New Windsor, NY) is a simple arrangement test consisting of 15 colored caps and one stationary reference cap (Figure 2-1). The test is quick and easy to administer. The colors are sufficiently distinct so that those with reduced visual acuity can usually see them, and young children can understand that they must make a "rainbow" out of the colors. The test provides easy differentiation between protan, deutan, and tritan defects. The patient is shown the caps (mixed up) and is asked to put the caps back in color order. After the patient has arranged the colors, the examiner flips the box over to reveal numbers on the underside of the caps (Figure 2-2). The numbers 1 through 15 and the reference cap form a circle on the score sheet. The numbers from the caps are then recorded on the score sheet in the order the patient has arranged them. The numbers are then connected by drawing lines (remember dot-to-dot puzzles?). If the patient made no errors, the numbers connect from 1 to 15 and form a circle on the test sheet (Figure 2-3). However, if the patient put the "15" cap next to the reference cap and the "1" cap next to the "15," the line would go from the refer-

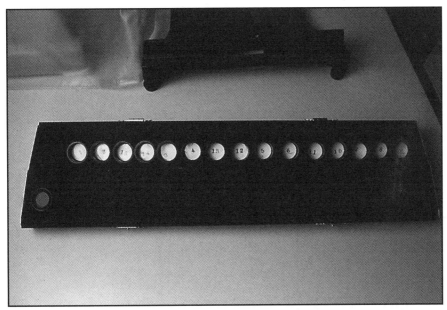

**Figure 2-2.** The underside of the D-15 Panel. The numbers are used to score the test. (Photograph by Ronald Morales.)

ence point to the 15, and then back to the 1 and so forth until all of the numbers had been connected. The way the patient arranges the caps reveals the type of defect present (Figures 2-4, 2-5, 2-6). The Farnsworth-Munsell D-15 Panel uses only saturated or brightly colored caps, therefore subtle defects, such as those seen in a mild anomalous trichromat, will not be detected.

### Desaturated 15 Panel

The Lanthony Desaturated 15 Panel (Luneau Ophtalmologie, Paris, France), uses a desaturated version of the Farnsworth-Munsell D-15 Panel. The colors in the desaturated version are extremely pale and are difficult to differentiate from white or from each other. This test is administered and scored identically to the Farnsworth-Munsell D-15 Panel. This test is also qualitative, but is very good at detecting subtle defects that may go unnoticed when the patient is tested using the Farnsworth-Munsell D-15 Panel.

### Farnsworth-Munsell 100-Hue Test

The most popular and the most time consuming arrangement test is the Farnsworth-Munsell 100-Hue Test (Munsell Division of GreytagMacBeth, New Windsor, NY). The test consists of 85 hues divided into four boxes, one with 22 caps and three with 21 caps (Figure 2-7). In each box are two stationary reference caps, one on each end. The patient is asked to arrange the colored caps from one box in a color order series between the two reference caps. The color caps are of equal lightness and are approximately equal in hue distance from one another. There is a subtle change in color from one cap to the next, and even some normal patients have difficulty differentiating certain caps. The caps compose a modified version of the full color spectrum and, when placed end-to-end, represent a color wheel.

Like the other arrangement tests, there is a number on the underside of each cap for determining the test score. The scoring technique is very different from the Farnsworth-Munsell D-15 Panel or the Lanthony Desaturated 15 panel, however. After the patient has completed the test,

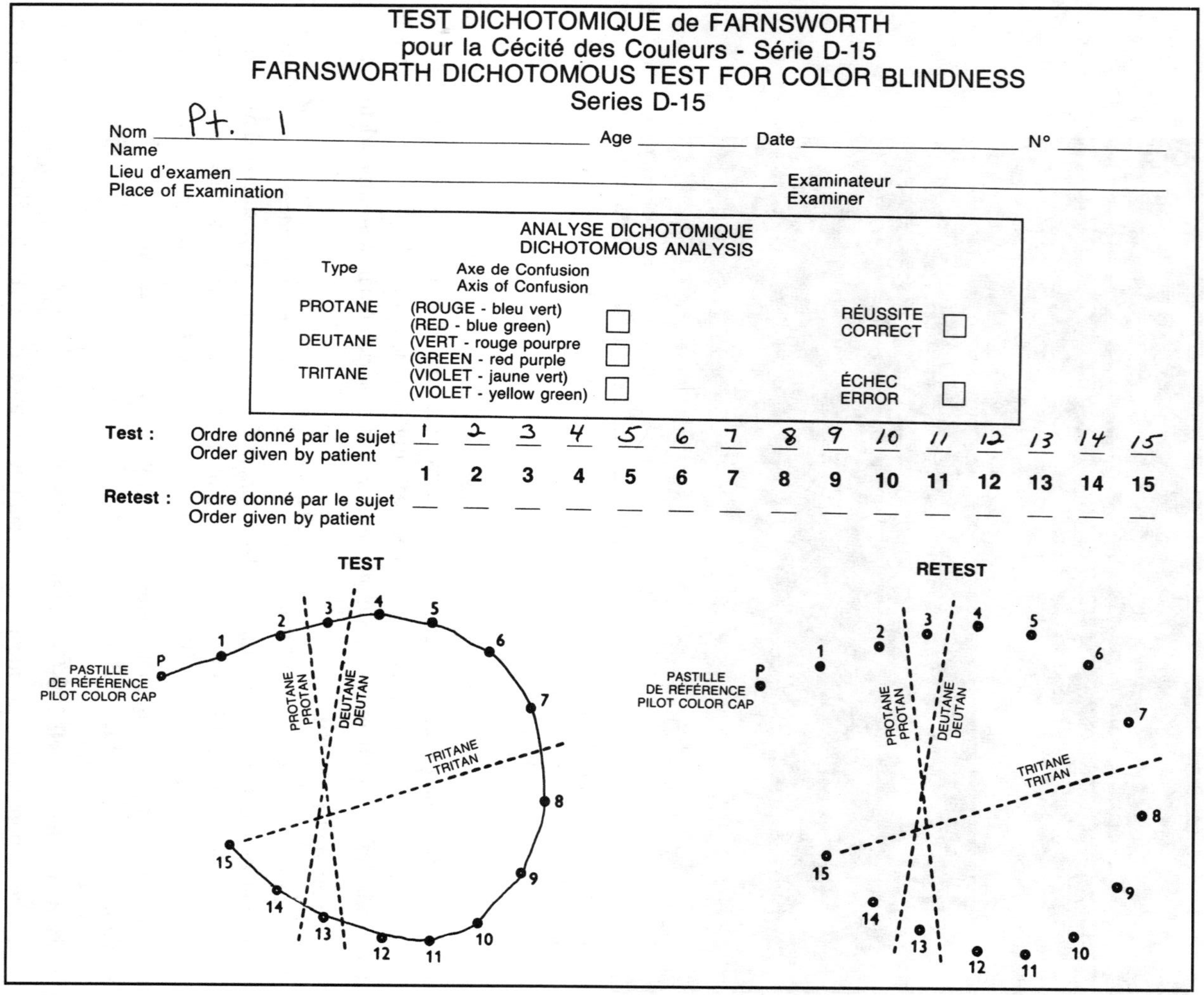
TEST DICHOTOMIQUE de FARNSWORTH
pour la Cécité des Couleurs - Série D-15
FARNSWORTH DICHOTOMOUS TEST FOR COLOR BLINDNESS
Series D-15

Nom / Name: Pt. 1 — Age ____ Date ____ N° ____

Lieu d'examen / Place of Examination ____ Examinateur / Examiner ____

ANALYSE DICHOTOMIQUE
DICHOTOMOUS ANALYSIS

| Type | Axe de Confusion / Axis of Confusion | |
|---|---|---|
| PROTANE | (ROUGE - bleu vert) (RED - blue green) | ☐ |
| DEUTANE | (VERT - rouge pourpre (GREEN - red purple | ☐ |
| TRITANE | (VIOLET - jaune vert) (VIOLET - yellow green) | ☐ |

RÉUSSITE / CORRECT ☐

ÉCHEC / ERROR ☐

| | | | | | | | | | | | | | | | | |
|---|---|---|---|---|---|---|---|---|---|---|---|---|---|---|---|---|
| Test : | Ordre donné par le sujet / Order given by patient | 1 | 2 | 3 | 4 | 5 | 6 | 7 | 8 | 9 | 10 | 11 | 12 | 13 | 14 | 15 |
| | | 1 | 2 | 3 | 4 | 5 | 6 | 7 | 8 | 9 | 10 | 11 | 12 | 13 | 14 | 15 |
| Retest : | Ordre donné par le sujet / Order given by patient | | | | | | | | | | | | | | | |



**Figure 2-3.** Results from a normal D-15 Panel.

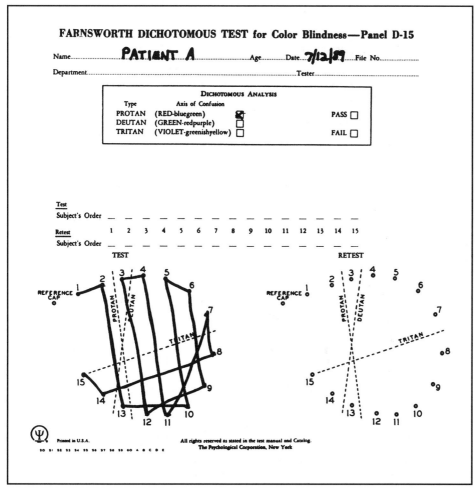

**Figure 2-4.** This D-15 scoresheet is typical of a protan defect. (Reprinted with permission from Benes SC, McKinney K, Sanders LC, Miller M, Moberg M. *Advanced Ophthalmic Diagnostics and Therapeutics*. Thorofare, NJ: SLACK Incorporated; 1990.)

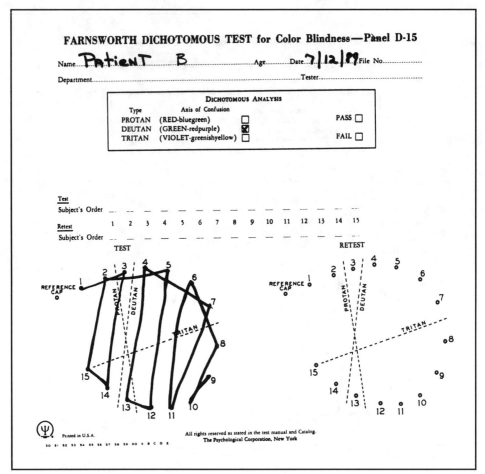

**Figure 2-5.** This D-15 scoresheet is typical of a deutan defect. (Reprinted with permission from Benes SC, McKinney K, Sanders LC, Miller M, Moberg M. *Advanced Ophthalmic Diagnostics and Therapeutics.* Thorofare, NJ: SLACK Incorporated; 1990.)

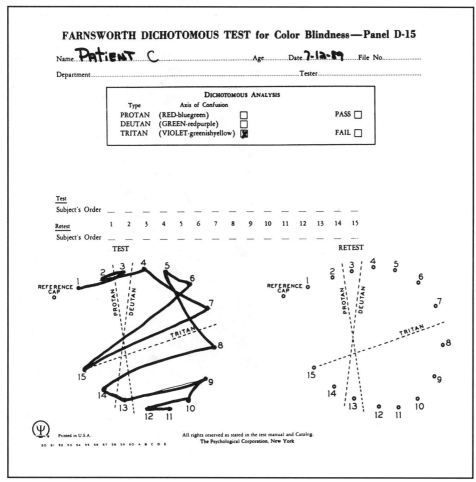

**Figure 2-6.** This D-15 scoresheet is typical of a tritan defect. (Reprinted with permission from Benes SC, McKinney K, Sanders LC, Miller M, Moberg M. *Advanced Ophthalmic Diagnostics and Therapeutics.* Thorofare, NJ: SLACK Incorporated; 1990.)

**Figure 2-7.** The Farnsworth-Munsell 100-Hue test. (Photograph by Ronald Morales.)

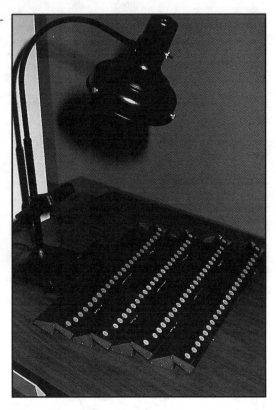

the examiner flips the box over and transcribes the patient's arrangement of the caps onto the test sheet (Figure 2-8).

In order to determine a particular score for a particular cap, we must look at the relationship of the cap to its adjacent neighbors. Suppose that a patient puts the first colored caps in this order: 3-4-6-5. The score for the cap in second place (4) is based on the absolute difference between cap 4 and its neighbor caps 3 and 6. To get the score for cap 4 we must subtract 4 from 3 (which equals 1) and 4 from 6 (which equals 2). (Remember we are looking for an absolute value, so the score will be 2 and not -2.) The 2 and the 1 are added together to give us a score of 3 for this cap. If the caps are in correct 1-2-3 order, the difference between 2 and 1 is 1 and the difference between 2 and 3 is 1. Therefore, the number 2 cap has a perfect score that is represented as 2. To get a final score, all of the cap errors are added together. Since 2 is a perfect score, it is not counted when the final scores are added together. Therefore a cap with a score of 4 actually has an error score of 2, since normal caps have a score of 2. Individuals with scores of greater than 100 are considered to have abnormal color vision. This number is based on a population average and may not be appropriate for very young children or for individuals with reduced visual acuity.

The patient's arrangement of the caps indicates the type of color mechanism involved. The original score for each cap is plotted on the score sheet. The score sheet is arranged in a circle. The examiner finds the score for cap 1 and places a dot on the corresponding location on the score sheet. If the score is 2, the dot will be on the innermost circle (meaning a perfect score). If the cap has a large score, such as 10, the examiner places a dot for that cap at the 10 circle. This suggests that the patient has extreme difficulty differentiating colors in this portion of the color wheel. This process of marking the score sheet is continued until all of the scores have been placed on the sheet. The dots are then connected to reveal the type of defect present. Very few

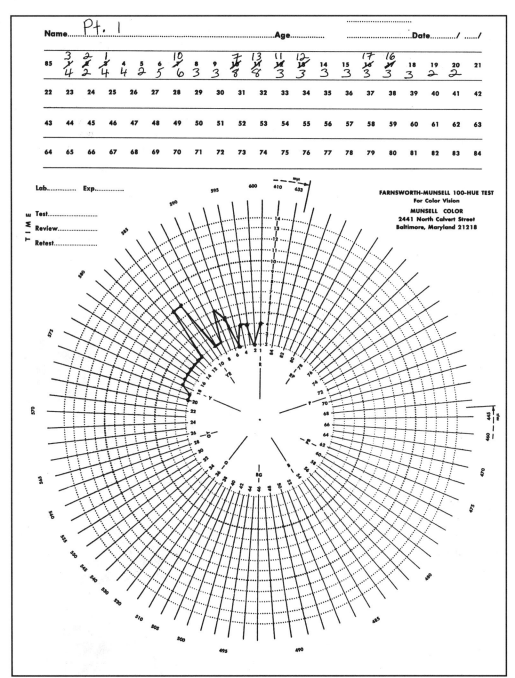

**Figure 2-8.** The score sheet from the Farnsworth-Munsell 100-Hue test. Patient responses are transcribed onto the score sheet and the numeric value for each cap is calculated based on the relationship of each cap to its two adjacent caps. The numeric value is then used to create a plot for the 100-Hue test.

**Figure 2-9.** Plot of a normal Farnsworth-Munsell 100-Hue test. Note that there is little deviation away from the inner circle. The inner circle represents a perfect relationship of the caps to their adjacent caps, thus signaling normal color perception. (Reprinted with permission from Jimenez-Sierra JM, Ogden TE, Van Boemel GB. *Inherited Retinal Diseases: A Diagnostic Guide.* St. Louis, Mo: CV Mosby Co.; 1989.)

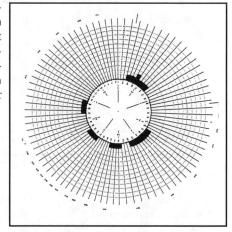

**Figure 2-10.** Plot of a Farnsworth-Munsell 100-Hue test showing a protan (red) defect. (Reprinted with permission from Jimenez-Sierra JM, Ogden TE, Van Boemel GB. *Inherited Retinal Diseases: A Diagnostic Guide.* St. Louis, Mo: CV Mosby Co.; 1989.)

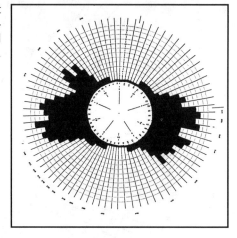

**Figure 2-11.** Plot of a Farnsworth-Munsell 100-Hue test showing a deutan (green) defect. (Reprinted with permission from Jimenez-Sierra JM, Ogden TE, Van Boemel GB. *Inherited Retinal Diseases: A Diagnostic Guide.* St. Louis, Mo: CV Mosby Co.; 1989.)

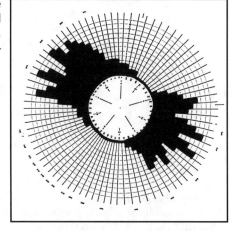

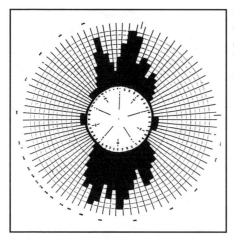

**Figure 2-12.** Plot of a Farnsworth-Munsell 100-Hue test showing a tritan (blue/yellow) defect. (Reprinted with permission from Jimenez-Sierra JM, Ogden TE, Van Boemel GB. *Inherited Retinal Diseases: A Diagnostic Guide.* St. Louis, Mo: CV Mosby Co.; 1989.)

errors and no axis of confusion (explained next) suggests normal color vision. A defect can represent a protan, deutan, tritan, or non-specific color vision defect (Figures 2-9 through 2-12).

The axis of confusion signifies the colors on the color wheel that are confused. In the protan defect, red and blue-green are confused. This means that colors on the opposite side of the color wheel are seen similarly, and may be placed next to one another (as was seen on the D-15 Panel score sheet). On the 100-Hue Test, the protan axis runs along a horizontal axis, the tritan axis runs along a vertical axis, and the deutan axis is between the protan and tritan axes (see Figures 2-10, 2-11, and 2-12).

## Color Matching Tests  The Anomaloscope

The arrangement tests are all qualitative; they reveal the type of defect, but not the severity of the defect. The anomaloscope, on the other hand, provides us with quantitative data on the severity of a particular defect. The most commonly used anomaloscopes test red/green abnormalities. There are anomaloscopes that test blue/yellow defects, but they are used only in research settings.

The patient is asked to look down the barrel of this elaborate test device (Figure 2-13), where he or she sees a colored circle. The circle may be all yellow, half red and half yellow, or half green and half yellow. The examiner manipulates the color of half of the circle, which ranges in color from green through yellow and through to red. The examiner creates a mixture of red and green and asks the patient if he or she can match the yellow half of the circle with the red/green color mixture by moving the yellow control knob (Figure 2-14). (The patient generally does not have control over the red/green control knob, but can be allowed to move both knobs if no perfect matches have been obtained in any other way.) Depending on how the examiner changes the red/green mixture, the color may look green, yellow-green, yellow, red-yellow, or red. For the normal individual, there is a very small range where the mixture of red and green appears yellow and therefore can be matched to the yellow test target. The normal person is very sensitive to slightly too much green, which makes the color look yellow/green, or to slightly too much red, which makes the color appear orange. Therefore the matching range for those with normal color vision is very small. For the patient with a red or green color vision defect, he (generally males have this problem) might need more green in his color to match yellow, as is the case in those with a deutan color defect. Conversely, the patient might need more red in the mixed color to match a yellow test target, as in the case of a person with a protan defect. The size of the match-

**Figure 2-13.** Patient seated at the anomaloscope. (Photograph by Ronald Morales.)

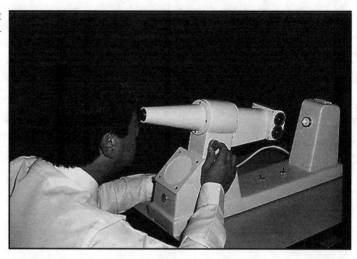

ing range determines if the defect is mild, moderate, severe, or absolute. If the matching range is only slightly enlarged and is more on the green side, we can state that the patient has a mild deutan or deuteranomalous defect. A larger range that goes from yellow to pure red, indicates that the patient has a moderate protan or protanamolous defect. The dichromatic patient with either an absolute green or red defect will be able to match pure spectral green with yellow as well as pure spectral red with yellow, and will match yellow with all the colors in between.

The intensity of the yellow color can also be manipulated by the patient, and this information can be useful in diagnosis. Individuals with protan defects will match pure spectral green with a light yellow; and pure spectral red with a very dark yellow (nearly black in color), as those with protan defects see red as black. Individuals with deutan defects will use the same intensity of yellow when matching green or red. Therefore, the difference in intensities of yellow used by patients when performing this test can be used to differentiate individuals with complete protan defects from those with complete deutan defects.

## What the Patient Needs to Know

- This is a test to check your color vision. Each eye will be tested separately.
- Please look down this tube. Can you see a colored circle?
- I control the color on the bottom half of the circle, and you control the color on the top half of the circle.
- Please look at this white light on the front of the device first.
- When I ask, I would like you to look down the tube and move this knob until the top and bottom half of the circle matches.
- The two halves must match perfectly. If they do not, tell me "no match."
- Then I want you to tell me why they do not match.
- We will repeat these steps until a matching range has been established for each of your eyes.
- This test will take about 20 minutes to perform.

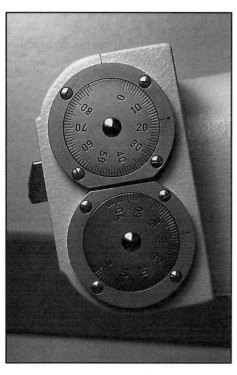

**Figure 2-14.** The top dial on this anomaloscope represents different intensities of yellow, ranging from a very pale yellow to near black (0). Yellow is generally controlled by the patient, who dials in the color using a knob on the opposite side of the unit. The bottom dial represents colors ranging from pure spectral green (number "0" on the dial) to pure spectral red (number "74" on the dial). The green/red mixture is controlled by the examiner. The patient is asked to match the yellow color with the green/red mixture (certain red/green combinations make yellow). The matching range is based on the dial's numeric values. The matching range determines if the person has normal or abnormal color vision. (Photograph by Ronald Morales.)

### Testing With the Anomaloscope

OptA

The patient is tested with one eye at a time. The patient should not be dilated, and may need spectacle correction. (Spectacle correction with this test is not as essential as it is with arrangement tests.) The patient is then shown a white light on the base of the unit, which "bleaches" the retina slightly. The patient is next instructed to look down the barrel and turn a knob on the unit to match the red/green mixture. The patient is again "bleached" while the examiner changes the red/green mixture dial to a new setting (see Figure 2-14). By doing this repeatedly, the examiner can determine the patient's matching range. If the patient is unable to make a perfect match between the red/green mixture and the yellow, the examiner notes the reason. Typical answers may be "too much red" or "too much green" in the color presented by the examiner. The examiner needs to make sure that the match is a perfect match and not just close. If a close match is recorded as perfect, this will artificially widen the final matching range and a normal individual may be given an inappropriate diagnosis of a slight color vision defect (Table 2-2).

## Dark Adaptometry

Dark adaptometry is a psychophysical test used to determine the ability of the rod photoreceptors to increase their sensitivity in the dark. In other words, the test is used to determine how well a person dark-adapts over time. For example, if you've been reading outside on a bright day and then go indoors, everything seems dim for about 5 minutes. This is because the rods and cones were "bleached" by the light and must adapt when you go inside.

Dark adaptometry is a useful test for anyone complaining of night vision problems. Test information can supplement the results obtained from other tests, such as the ERG and EOG (see Chapters 6 and 7). If the patient is cooperative, the results will provide excellent information as

Table 2-2.

## Anomaloscope Readings Showing the Normal Range and Abnormal Ranges for Protan and Deutan Defects

Anomaloscope readings showing the normal range and abnormal ranges for protan and deutan defects.[296]

| NORMAL TRICHROMATIC VISION | PROTAN DEFECTS | DEUTAN DEFECTS |
|---|---|---|
| Range: 37 to 45 | **Protanopia (Intensity Matching Abnormal,† Farnsworth-Munsell 100-Hue Protan Axis)**<br>Range: 0 to 73 | **Deuteranopia (Intensity Matching Normal,† Farnsworth-Munsell 100-Hue Deutan Axis)**<br>Range: 0 to 73 |
| **Probably Normal: Slightly Altered Equation**<br>Wide equation: 39 to 49<br>Less wide equation: 41 to 48<br>Wide equation shift to red end: 40 to 50<br>Wide equation shift to green end: 35 to 45<br>Wide equation shift to both ends: 35 to 50 | **Protanomalous Defect—Mild**<br>Protanomalous defect: narrow equation: 45 to 50<br>Protanomalous defect: wide equation: 41 to 55<br>Slight protanomalous defect: equation: 42 to 55<br>Slight protanomalous defect: wide equation: 41 to 57 | **Deuteranomalous Defect—Mild**<br>Deuteranomalous defect: mild: 20 to 30 |
| | **Protanomalous Defect—Moderate to Severe**<br>Protanomalous defect: mild to moderate: 40 to 57<br>Protanomalous defect: moderate: 50 to 73<br>Protanomalous defect: moderate to severe: 25 to 73 | **Deuteranomalous Defect—Moderate**<br>Deuteranomalous defect: mild to moderate (narrow equation): 10 to 20<br>Deuteranomalous defect: mild to moderate: 6 to 30<br>Deuteranomalous defect: moderate: 0 to 25<br>Deuteranomalous defect: moderate: 0 to 30 |

*(Reprinted with permission from Jimenez-Sierra JM, Ogden TE, Van Boemel GB. Inherited Retinal Diseases: A Diagnostic Guide. St. Louis, Mo: CV Mosby Co.; 1989.)*

## What the Patient Needs to Know

- Dark adaptometry is a test to check how well you see in the dark.
- The test is lasts about 45 minutes.
- We will first sit in the dark for 2 minutes. Then you will put your chin in the chin rest of the apparatus, and keep your eyes wide open.
- There will be a bright background light. This bright light will get your eyes ready to be tested in the dark.
- After you have been exposed to the bright light for 5 minutes, the light will be turned off and you will be in total darkness.
- You will be asked to tell the examiner just as soon as you are able to see a very dim light from behind the test target at the back of the bowl. You will be tested with this target over and over again for at least 30 minutes.

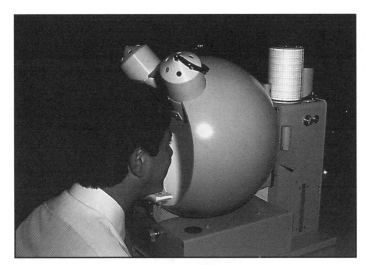

**Figure 2-15.** A patient seated at the Goldmann-Weekers dark adaptometer. (Photograph by Ronald Morales.)

to how well he or she sees in the dark, compared to a normal population. There may be subtle changes in night vision that are easily detected by this test that cannot be detected by means of the electroretinogram. The test is generally performed with the Goldmann-Weekers dark adaptometer. The dark adaptometer resembles a Goldmann perimeter in shape but not in function (Figure 2-15).

## Administering the Test

The patient is given instructions on what is expected of him or her during the test. Initially, the patient is dark-adapted for 2 minutes. After the 2 minute period, the patient is light-adapted for 5 minutes. The adaptation light is in the dark adaptometry bowl. The patient places his or her head in a chin rest and is instructed to keep his or her eyes open while looking straight ahead in the illuminated bowl. This is a crucial part of the test, as it results in the "bleaching" of the rod and cone pigments, thus resulting in both rod and cone adaptation.

Once the patient has watched the bright background light for 5 minutes, all of the lights are turned off, leaving the patient in virtual darkness. The patient is asked to look straight ahead and report when he or she sees a very dim test target. The test target is a translucent piece of plastic with black bars painted on it, that lies over a light at the back of the adaptometer bowl (Figure 2-16). When the light is turned on it shines through the target and the patient sees either three white bars or two black bars. The intensity of the light is controlled by the examiner. When the patient reports seeing the bars, the examiner marks the score sheet and turns the target light completely off. The examiner repeats the process about once every 30 seconds for 30 minutes. In cases where the patient has normal night vision, the individual should be able to see dimmer and dimmer targets as time elapses.

After the first 5 minutes of dark adaptation, the patient is asked to fixate on a small red light that is about 2 inches above the fixation light. The patient is instructed to continue fixing on the red light, while still reporting when he or she first sees the bars of the test target. By having the patient fixate at this level, the rod-rich area of the retina is tested.

The score sheet is attached to a slowly rotating drum. To increase target intensity, the examiner rotates a knob on the side of the unit that is calibrated in log units of light. As the knob is

**Figure 2-16.** The inside of the Goldmann-Weekers dark adaptometer. The opaque black bars are painted on top of a translucent white disk. After the lights have been extinguished, the examiners brings up a very dim light that back-illuminates the white disk. Patients see either white bars or black bars (based on perception) and are asked to inform the examiner as soon as the bars are barely visible. (Photograph by Ronald Morales.)

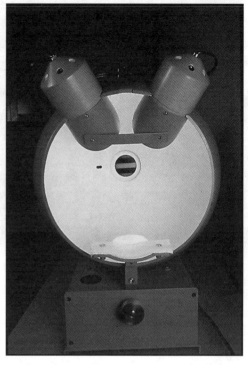

rotated, the light behind the target increases in intensity. The light intensity is also shown by a line on a vertically numbered light strip (the larger the number, the brighter the light) (Figure 2-17). As the light increases in intensity, the line on the light strip moves up. The line corresponds to an arm that is next to the rotating drum. As the line goes up, so does the arm. When the patient sees the dim light, the score sheet on the drum is marked by a pin on the arm. (The examiner moves the knob forward, which makes the arm move toward the drum.) At the end of the test, the little pinpricks on the score sheet are connected in "connect-the-dot" fashion. The score sheet represents the level of light intensity seen over time.

## Evaluating the Dark Adaptometry Curve

Figure 2-18 shows a normal dark adaptometry curve. Initially the patient was only able to see a very bright light (remember, the greater the number, the brighter the light), but as time progressed was able to see a dimmer and dimmer light. At the end of 30 minutes, the normal eye is about 80% dark-adapted. This is manifested by the patient being able to see light at the $10^2$ log unit level. This is referred to as the final rod threshold, which is normal in this patient (see Figure 2-18, Label B). The normal final rod threshold suggests that the patient sees 100,000 times better in the dark at the end of the test than he or she did after the light was first extinguished. The figure shows a short, quick curve followed by a slower curve. The quick curve represents cone adaptation, whereas the slow, second curve represents rod adaptation. The intersection of the two curves (see Figure 2-18, Label A) is known as the rod/cone break. Initially, cones are responsible for the adaptation because of the bright background light that the patient observed for 5 minutes before the test started (comparable to the adaptation you notice coming inside after reading outdoors). After about 5 minutes, the cones are no longer able to continue to dark-adapt, since

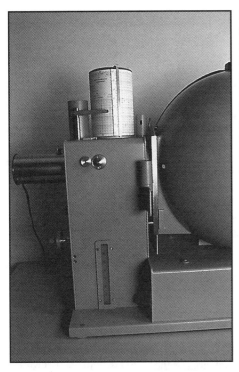

**Figure 2-17.** The side of the Goldmann-Weekers dark adaptometer where the examiner controls the intensity of light that back-illuminates the white disk. The light intensity corresponds to log units of light, with the lower numbers corresponding to dimmer light. A knob is turned by the examiner. This knob controls both the level of illumination and also a small bar that protrudes next to the rotating drum. As the patient reports seeing the dim light, the examiner pulls the knob forward, thus piercing the score sheet on the rotating drum. (Photograph by Ronald Morales.)

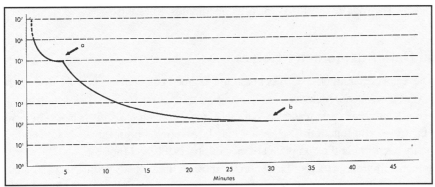

**Figure 2-18.** A normal dark adaptometry curve. Note the first rapidly descending curve on the left. This represents cone adaptation. After about five minutes, the cones no longer dark adapt, but the rods start to dark adapt. This is known as the rod/cone break and is depicted by label A. The rods slowly dark adapt (note the slow descending curve after the rod/cone break) to a final rod threshold that is 3 log units below the cone threshold (label B). (Reprinted with permission from Jimenez-Sierra JM, Ogden TE, Van Boemel GB. *Inherited Retinal Diseases: A Diagnostic Guide.* St. Louis, Mo: CV Mosby Co.; 1989.)

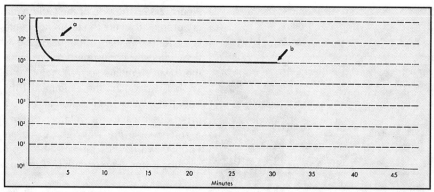

**Figure 2-19.** An abnormal dark adaptometry curve, showing a normal cone curve and a complete absence of a rod curve. This pattern would be seen in individuals who have a virtual absence of rod function, such as individuals with retinitis pigmentosa. (Reprinted with permission from Jimenez-Sierra JM, Ogden TE, Van Boemel GB. *Inherited Retinal Diseases: A Diagnostic Guide.* St. Louis, Mo: CV Mosby Co.; 1989.)

cones do not perceive dim light very well. It is the rods that affect continued dark adaptation. During the phase when the rods are tested for adaptation ability, the patient is looking at the red fixation light in the bowl. This assures that the most rod-rich area of the retina is being tested for its ability to dark-adapt. The rods adapt slowly over the 30 minutes of testing.

## Abnormal Dark Adaptometry Curves

Those who have abnormal night vision, as in retinitis pigmentosa, will not be able to see better in the dark over time. We can measure this by using dark adaptometry The dark adaptometry in Figure 2-19 shows a normal cone response, but there is no "rod curve." This is a very typical pattern where there is no rod function. The person may have retinitis pigmentosa or some other type of abnormality resulting in the complete absence of observable rod function.

Dark adaptometry findings will also be abnormal in those individuals with abnormal cone function. In Figure 2-20 there is no "cone curve." This pattern is frequently seen in individuals who have very poorly functioning cones, such as those with cone dystrophy or rod monochromatism. In this case only the rods function, and they do not respond quickly when first exposed to the dark.

If the dark adaptometry curve does not look fairly similar to the one in Figure 2-18, we can assume that the results are abnormal. An abnormal curve may represent abnormal rod function as in Figure 2-19, or abnormal cone function as in Figure 2-20. The curve may also look abnormal due to poor patient cooperation. It is important to distinguish true pathology from feigned abnormality. A patient who is malingering may have an abnormal dark adaptometry examination, but the person's responses will be very inconsistent (Figure 2-21). Such inconsistencies are not seen in those with true pathology, and therefore support a diagnosis of malingering. It is important that such inconsistencies are reported to the doctor ordering the test.

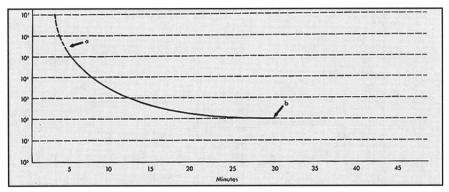

**Figure 2-20.** An abnormal dark adaptometry curve, showing a normal rod curve and an abnormal cone curve and absence of the rod/cone break. This pattern would be seen in individuals with abnormally functioning cones, such as those with cone dystrophy. (Reprinted with permission from Jimenez-Sierra JM, Ogden TE, Van Boemel GB. *Inherited Retinal Diseases: A Diagnostic Guide.* St. Louis, Mo: CV Mosby Co.; 1989.)

## Points to Remember When Administering the Test

Dark adaptometry is a very simple test to administer. The patient can be dilated, but this can cause discomfort and the patient is likely to close his or her eyes during light adaptation. If that occurs, then the cone curve and the rod/cone break might be erroneously abnormal.

The patient is instructed to report when he or she can just barely see the light. Some individuals will wait until they can see the light fairly well before informing the examiner. This is generally obvious to the examiner, since the patient's results will not be consistent. When the patient is reporting exactly when he or she first distinguishes the light, there will be very little inconsistency in responses between trials.

It is advisable to set the height of the adaptometer and chin rest prior to the initial 2 minute dark adaptation period. You might allow the patient to sit away from the bowl during this dark adaptation phase. When it is time to light-adapt the patient, you can ask the individual to find the chin rest with his or her hand and then lean forward into it. If the adaptometer bowl is not in the proper position, you will need to adjust it during the light phase. This is awkward and should be avoided.

Do not increase the test light too quickly. It is possible to falsely elevate a final rod threshold by making the light brighten too quickly. The patient will not be able to respond quickly enough, and by the time he or she reports seeing the light, the intensity of the light is significantly greater. (This is very similar to presenting the test target too quickly while doing Goldmann perimetry. In that case, the patient's visual fields will be artificially constricted. In the case of dark adaptometry testing, the final rod threshold will be artificially elevated.)

When conducting the test, you must provide your own timing device. A red illuminated stopwatch works best. The red face is easily seen by the examiner and should not interfere with the test.

This is a very long examination, and some patients may need to stop and stretch during the test. This is perfectly acceptable, but should be done after about 15 minutes of testing when the most critical portion of the test (the quick cone adaptation curve and cone/rod break) is completed. For the most part the patient should remain still during the examination.

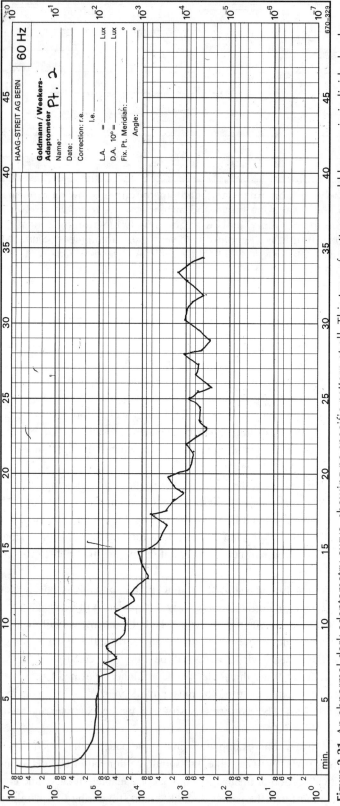

**Figure 2-21.** An abnormal dark adaptometry curve, showing no specific pattern at all. This type of pattern would be seen in individuals who are malingering since it is impossible for the individual to "know" exactly what intensity of light they responded to previously. This is similar in concept to crossing isopters in a Goldmann visual field test.

Finally, it is absolutely essential that the room be light-tight, similar to a photographic dark-room. Any light in the room, including lights from telephones, etc, may reduce the patient's ability to perceive very dim light. The room light might be brighter than the dim lights you are testing for, resulting in artificially elevated final rod thresholds.

# The Macular Photostress Test

The macular photostress test determines how quickly vision recovers after an individual has been exposed to bright light. Remember for a moment how your vision is reduced after seeing an oncoming car that has its bright headlights on. This sensation of reduced visual acuity is common to all individuals after exposure to very bright light; however, the sensation of reduced vision can be prolonged in those individuals who have macular disease. This vision decrease is caused by the temporary bleaching of the retina as a result of exposure to a very bright light. Visual recovery occurs as the visual pigments in the photoreceptors are resynthesized. In patients with macular disease, the resynthesis period is prolonged due to abnormality of the retinal pigment epithelium (RPE) in the macular area. This test is useful even in very early macular disease.

This test can also be quite useful in differentiating between macular and optic nerve pathology. There is no abnormality in the photoreceptor outer segments or the RPE in those individuals who have optic nerve disease. Therefore, those with optic nerve disease should have normal results on this test.

Normal individuals should be tested to develop a normal response range for comparison with the tested patients. Testing about 20 people should produce a reliable normal range.

## Administering the Test

The patient should be seated in a dimly lit exam room. The patient's best vision should be documented prior to beginning the test. The examiner shines a bright light, either from a transilluminator or direct ophthalmoscope, into one of the patient's eyes for 10 seconds. The other eye should be covered. The light is then extinguished and the patient is asked to read the eye chart at one line above their best vision (ie, read the 20/25 line if vision is 20/20) as soon as the vision has recovered enough to do so. For the average patient it takes about 30 seconds to recover from exposure to the bright light before being able to read the eye chart again. For most individuals with normal vision, recovery should occur in less than 50 seconds after the light is extinguished. The recovery time is noted for one eye, and then the other eye is tested in a similar manner. There should be very little difference between the two eyes. If there is significant difference in recovery time between the two eyes (more than 20 seconds), there may be unequal pathology present or early pathology in the eye with a prolonged recovery time.

Documentation of the results should include the patient's best visual acuity, the Snellen line read after light exposure (one line above best visual acuity), and the amount of time that elapsed between exposure and the patient being able to read that line. Normal values for that particular clinic also should be noted. The results might look like this:

*Macular photostress test (10 second exposure)*
*(BVA = best visual acuity)*

Clinic normal = 40 secs

OD                BVA cc 20/60; 20/70 in 310 seconds

OS                BVA cc 20/40; 20/50 in 110 seconds

This method of recording the results clearly indicates the best visual acuity, the tested acuity, and the recovery time. Progression of any abnormality can be noted as visual acuity and recovery time changes over the course of the disease.

# The Potential Acuity Meter

In an ideal world, every patient who came in for an eye examination would have perfectly clear media and a readily-diagnosable problem. In such patients, visual acuity would be easy to determine. However, we must often estimate a patient's visual potential when his or her media are not clear. Estimating visual potential may be very important, especially in an eye that has both opaque media and a history of such problems as trauma or macular degeneration. Prior to cataract surgery on an eye that might not regain normal visual acuity, an estimate of postoperative potential is recommended. Such estimates are generally obtained using a device called the Potential Acuity Meter (PAM) (Marco Ophthalmic Co, Jacksonville, Fla).

The PAM is a portable device that is attached to the very front of the slit lamp (Figure 2-22). There are two light sources on the PAM. One is red and the other looks like a small white light. The white light is actually a miniature acuity chart which is projected onto the patient's retina. This brightly illuminated acuity chart is approximately 0.15 mm in diameter. Like most other acuity charts, the larger letters are on the top. The smallest letters correspond to a 20/20 equivalent and are denoted by the number 9. Unlike an eye chart used in the clinic, this chart is so small and bright that it can be shown through small clear areas of the cataract (or media opacity). There are some instances when either the cataract or media opacity is too dense for this test to work successfully, but in many cases there is a small area where the light can pass through. It is essential that the patient be dilated for this test to maximize the area through which the image can shine on the retina.

The patient is asked to place his or her forehead against the bar with his or her chin in the chin rest. The patient's spherical equivalent refraction is dialed in by rotating a knob on the side of the unit. The spherical units are displayed horizontally on the side of the PAM that faces the examiner (Figure 2-23). Once the patient's prescription has been dialed in, the actual examination can begin.

The red light is shown into the patient's eye and the patient is asked whether or not the red light is visible. The room light is then turned off. Then the white light is shown to the patient, and again, the patient is asked whether or not the white light is seen (Figure 2-24). The examiner must make sure that the white light is over the pupil. Once the white light has been properly aligned over the patient's pupil, the patient is asked what is seen. If the patient reports seeing letters, then he or she is asked to read them from the top of the chart down. The PAM letters are printed on the side of the unit for easy reference (Figure 2-25). If the patient reports seeing a white light but no letters, it may be because the chart is not in proper focus. Have the

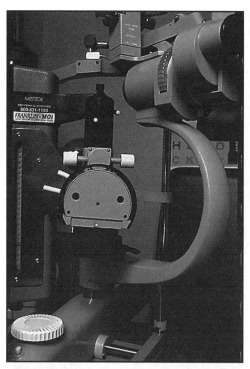

**Figure 2-22.** The PAM mounted to a slit lamp. (Photograph by Nilo Davila.)

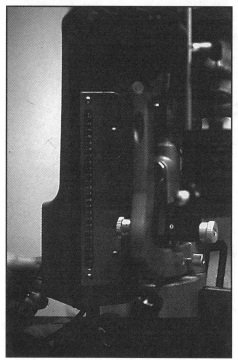

**Figure 2-23.** Set the sliding scale for the spherical refraction to the patient's distance refraction. (Reprinted with permission from Benes SC, McKinney K, Sanders LC, Miller M, Moberg M. *Advanced Ophthalmic Diagnostics and Therapeutics.* Thorofare, NJ: SLACK Incorporated; 1990.)

**Figure 2-24.** Instruct the patient to observe the red illuminating light. Then turn off the room lights and allow him or her to adapt to the darkness. (Reprinted with permission from Benes SC, McKinney K, Sanders LC, Miller M, Moberg M. *Advanced Ophthalmic Diagnostics and Therapeutics.* Thorofare, NJ: SLACK Incorporated; 1990.)

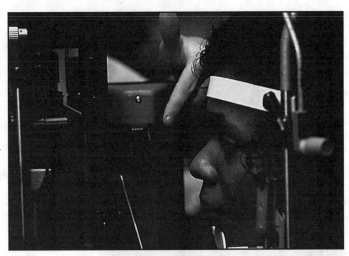

**Figure 2-25.** Follow the chart along with the patient as he or she reads down it. Record the patient's best PAM acuity for each eye. (Reprinted with permission from Benes SC, McKinney K, Sanders LC, Miller M, Moberg M. *Advanced Ophthalmic Diagnostics and Therapeutics.* Thorofare, NJ: SLACK Incorporated; 1990.)

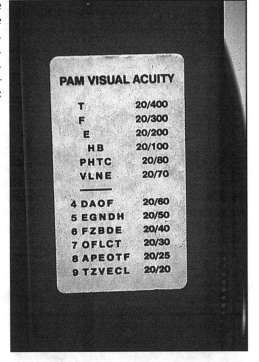

patient rotate the spherical equivalent knob until the letters become clear. If it does not become clear, move the light source for the chart slightly, and ask patient to try again. If after several tries, moving the instrument and/or readjustment of the spherical correction does not enable the patient to see the chart, discontinue the test. Testing the patient's better eye first may be advisable, so that the patient will see the chart better and have a general idea of what is expected during the test.

Care should be taken when testing the patient, as any head movement will move the chart. Patients can be told to clench the jaws while reading to reduce head movement. Likewise, the chin rest can be lowered out of the way once the patient has been properly positioned. It may be advisable to have the patient only read two letters per line until the last line is seen, to reduce the potential of head movement and image displacement.

Document the patient's PAM vision in a manner similar to that of a regular visual acuity exam, but indicate that the vision was obtained using the PAM. If the patient does not see any of the letters, indicate in the chart that the PAM was unsuccessfully attempted. Write something like "PAM—Unable, OU."

The PAM visual acuity test should give the physician and the patient a general idea of postoperative visual acuity. Certainly this examination does not guarantee that the person's vision will be at the tested level. There may be unforeseen complications during surgery, but there may also be other reasons for poor predictions. The area of retina that is tested with the PAM is very small. Because of that, if there is widespread damage with some normal retina remaining, the area tested may represent the normal retina. If that is the case, the patient may have significant metamorphopsia postoperatively that was not detected using the tiny PAM chart. Overall, the PAM is a useful tool in estimating visual potential in many eyes with opacified media.

## The Glare Test and the Brightness Acuity Test*

Frequently, individuals with early cataracts who do not have significantly reduced vision will still complain of serious problems with glare. Such individuals may be very visually limited, while at the same time have relatively normal standard visual acuity. This is due to the fact that the opacities scatter the light coming into the eye in many directions, resulting in brightness of vision but not clarity. Also, each opacity will have a different index of refraction, further reducing the clarity. In such cases, the ophthalmologist may want to demonstrate that the patient is visually debilitated by these mild opacities (such as posterior subcapsular cataracts) and that these opacities result in significant glare. Such documentation may result in the approval of cataract surgery by an insurance company in an eye with only a mild cataract.

There are several different devices that can be used to assess the effects of glare on vision. In this section, two types of tests will be reviewed: the glare test and the Brightness Acuity Test (BAT) (Marco Ophthalmic Co, Jacksonville, Fla).

### Standard Glare Testing

The standard glare test is done easily in the ophthalmology office and does not require any special equipment. It is not as precise as the BAT, but should be useful in documenting visual disability due to glare. Initially, the patient is tested using a Snellen chart in a darkened room with his or her best spectacle correction, one eye at a time. The patient's vision is noted and identified as being taken in a darkened environment by writing the word "dimness" next to the acuity. Again the patient is tested, but this time with the room lights on. Acuities are noted in the chart and labeled "room lighting" to identify that the acuities were obtained when the room lights were on. The patient is finally tested with the room lights on and an additional light entering the eye. The additional light is generally obtained using a transilluminator that is directed into the patient's eye at approximately a 20 degree angle horizontal to the pupil (Figure 2-26). Again, each eye is tested separately and the acuity recorded, but the word "brightness" is used to denote the conditions under which the test was performed.

**Figure 2-26.** The third stage of glare testing requires that the patient be tested using light in addition to standard room lighting. This is accomplished by shining light from a transilluminator into the patient's eye while the patient is reading the eye chart. The transilluminator is angled 20 degrees horizontal to the pupil. (Photograph by Nilo Davila.)

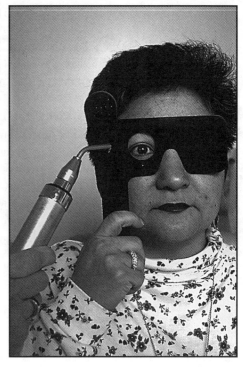

In patients who have little problem with glare, vision will be approximately the same under all three lighting conditions. In those who have problems with glare, vision will be fairly good under "dim" conditions, but will worsen with increasing amounts of light. The person who has significant problems with glare may be unable to read anything smaller than the 20/200 letter under "bright" conditions. Because of the ease of administering this test, it can be done on virtually every patient who complains of problems with glare. However, different vision charts may need to be used to reduce the possibility of memorization.

## Brightness Acuity Testing

In the event that more precise control of the lighting conditions is necessary, the Brightness Acuity Test can be performed. This is a battery-charged instrument that looks like a miniature perimeter attached to a direct ophthalmoscope handle (Figure 2-27). The beauty of this device is that it standardizes the lighting conditions, thus allowing for accurate follow-up of patients over time. The BAT has a light source that can be adjusted and a 12 mm opening for peering at the Snellen chart. The test is conducted in a similar manner to the standard glare test. The patient is first tested with his or her best correction, one eye at a time, in a dimly lit room without the BAT. The acuity is documented and noted as being taken with the room lights off. The next three acuities are taken with the patient viewing through the BAT, which is held over the eye being examined. The other eye must be closed. Initially, the dial is set to "low." This setting mimics natural room light but standardizes it (unlike the standard glare test technique). Acuity is recorded and noted as being taken with the BAT setting at "low." The setting is then moved to "medium." This mimics sunlight at noon outdoors. The acuity is noted in the chart as indicated above. Finally, the setting is moved to "high." This represents a significant glare

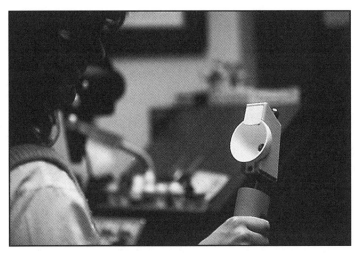

**Figure 2-27.** A BAT (Brightness Acuity Tester) has a 12 mm aperture through which the patient looks while wearing his or her best correction. The inside of the hemisphere rests over the eye. The matte white surface reflects light into the pupil from all directions. There are three brightness settings to produce glare. (Reprinted with permission from Benes SC, McKinney K, Sanders LC, Miller M, Moberg M. *Advanced Ophthalmic Diagnostics and Therapeutics.* Thorofare, NJ: SLACK Incorporated; 1990.)

effect and mimics bright sunlight being reflected off of white sand, snow, or concrete. This acuity is also noted in the chart. The results indicate visual acuities for each eye under four separate lighting conditions.

As with the standard glare test, those with problems that result from opacities will report decreasing visual acuity as the intensity of the BAT light increases. As is true with any special test, accurate documentation of the patient's complaints is essential and may result in the patient with a mild cataract being able to obtain surgery.

*The information in this section does not appear on the ophthalmic technology exam.*

# Contrast Sensitivity

Snellen-type visual acuity charts have been used since the mid-1800s, and are considered the standard method of evaluating visual acuity. These charts use high-contrast black letters and shapes of specified sizes on white backgrounds. Although this is a commonly used method for visual acuity testing, it may not adequately evaluate how well a person is actually able to see. Many individuals with essentially normal Snellen acuity, in the range of 20/40 or better, may complain of poor vision. They may report that objects appear as if viewed through fog, that their vision seems hazy, that colors do not seem sharp, and/or that glare is a significant problem. These individuals may have problems with contrast vision.

The problems with contrast can range from very mild to quite severe. These problems may be due to retinal or optic nerve abnormalities, cataracts, corneal scars, refractive errors, or contact lens use. The only way to evaluate these complaints is with contrast sensitivity tests.

Most individuals have normal contrast vision. However, even for those individuals with normal contrast vision, there is a point at which it is impossible to distinguish between objects that are only subtly different in contrast. For example, we all know how difficult it is to see a person dressed in dark clothing who crosses right in front of us while we are driving down a very dark street at night. It is not until the person is in our headlights that he or she becomes visible. That is because the individual is in a dimly lit environment of low contrast.

Conversely, there are also problems viewing objects of low contrast in a brightly-lit environment. For example, it may be difficult to view something white on a white sandy beach on a very sunny day. It may also be difficult to view something light-colored on a foggy day, and it may be virtually impossible to view streetlights on a foggy night. Everything appears washed out, colorless, and without contrast.

These are all situations in which an individual with normal contrast vision will have difficulty seeing. Individuals with poor contrast vision will find normal visual situations to be very visually challenging. It is for this reason that contrast sensitivity testing has become a very important addition to the standard Snellen-style acuity test. Therefore, anyone who complains of difficulty with vision should be tested using contrast sensitivity tests.

## Contrast Sensitivity Tests

Contrast sensitivity tests have been in existence for some time. In 1918, an ophthalmologist made what was probably the first contrast sensitivity test. He drew circular gratings (black and white or grey and white lines with blurred edges) in a book using more and more diluted ink to make the drawings. He asked his patients to identify the direction the gratings were pointing, noting the dimmest grating the patient was able to correctly identify. Contrast sensitivity tests have remained essentially the same since this first version.

The test comes in a variety of styles, but all of them have one thing in common. They consist of letters, objects, or gratings that are of graduated contrast. The tests are given in a similar manner in that the patient is asked to identify the faintest object or grating on the chart.

There are now several commercially available contrast sensitivity tests. These can be found on either charts or in computer systems like B-VAT (Mentor Ophthalmic Instruments, Norwell, MA). Some are similar to Snellen charts, with letters of varying shades of gray (instead of high-contrast black letters) (Figure 2-28). Some of the charts have light gray letters on white backgrounds, while others have dark gray letters on black backgrounds. Children's versions using Allen-type objects, tumbling E's, or faces are also available (Figure 2-29). (The face cards are often used in a fashion that is similar to preferential looking. The very young child will be shown either a white card or a card with a dim face on it. The dimmest face that the child responds to would represent the child's visual threshold. The level of contrast between each face is quite significant, therefore the test evaluates only gross contrast vision.) All of these tests provide gross estimates of contrast sensitivity.

There are more sophisticated forms of contrast sensitivity testing. Some use computer programs that display sinusoidal gratings of various contrasts and frequencies. Sinusoidal gratings are waves that go up and down evenly, with a dark trough and a light peak (Figure 2-30). The waves appear as fuzzy lines on the contrast sensitivity test. The patient is asked to identify the direction of the gratings. The gratings go either to the right, to the left, or straight up and down. There are also charts that use round disks containing sinusoidal gratings of various contrasts and frequencies; these are the most common types used in eyecare practices (Figure 2-31). The tests using the sinusoidal gratings are more sophisticated than the contrast sensitivity tests that use objects or letters, and provide more in-depth information on a person's ability to see contrast. The results provided by the tests using sinusoidal gratings are referred to as contrast sensitivity functions.

## Performing Contrast Sensitivity Testing

Like any visual acuity test, contrast sensitivity tests should be conducted with the patient's best spectacle correction and at the properly assigned distance. (Some tests are designed for near

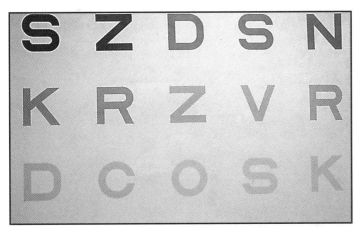

**Figure 2-28.** An ETDRS-style chart used for contrast sensitivity testing. (Photograph by Nilo Davila.)

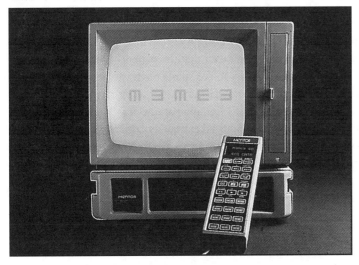

**Figure 2-29.** CRT screen contrast sensitivity tumbling E's. (Photo courtesy of Mentor O&O, Inc.)

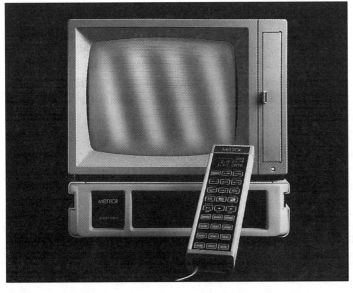

**Figure 2-30.** CRT sinuso bar gratings, this one ang left. (Photo courtesy of N tor O&O, Inc.)

**Figure 2-31.** Vistech contrast sensitivity chart. (Photograph by Nilo Davila.)

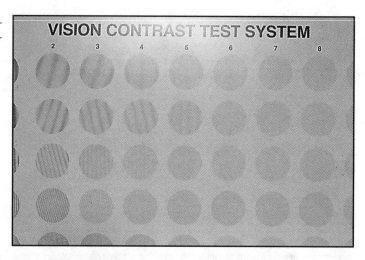

**Figure 2-31.** Vistech contrast sensitivity chart. (Photograph by Nilo Davila.)

testing, while others are designed for distance testing.) Visibility is a critical part of proper administration of contrast sensitivity tests. Care should be taken that the patient's glasses are not significantly tinted. (Tinting may reduce the eye's ability to see subtle contrasts. Provide the patient with his or her spectacle correction in a trial frame if necessary.)

Patients need to be tested using the manufacturer's lighting parameters. Some contrast sensitivity tests actually come with light meters, as lighting is an extremely critical component to contrast sensitivity testing. The tests have been calibrated using specific lighting conditions, and the normal and abnormal ranges have been developed based on these conditions. If a person is tested using the wrong lighting, the individual may appear to have abnormal contrast sensitivity when in fact the lighting was either too bright or not bright enough.

Each eye should be tested separately, with the better eye being tested first. The patient should be told that he or she will be viewing objects (or gratings) of various contrasts and to identify either the object or the direction the grating is pointing. Tell the patient that it is important to respond even when unsure about the correctness of the answer. (In other words, encourage the patient to guess when near his or her visual threshold.) If the patient reports seeing only the obvious objects and is not encouraged to guess at the less visible objects, then the visual threshold will be artificially elevated. Patients need to be told that everyone has difficulty seeing the very dim gratings or letters. Encourage the patient to continue until the responses are consistently wrong. The last correctly identified object, letter, or grating must be noted in the patient's chart. The contrast sensitivity charts that are similar to Snellen charts also use a similar notation (ie, 20/40), but the level of contrast that the patient needed in order to read the letters accurately must also be noted (ie, 40%). The level of contrast can be found on either the chart or on the computer remote control (see Figure 2-30).

Contrast sensitivity tests that use the sinusoidal gratings come with score sheets. These should be filled out completely and included in the patient's chart. The configuration of the patient's responses to the contrast sensitivity gratings results in the contrast sensitivity function. A contrast sensitivity function indicates whether the patient's contrast vision is normal or abnormal, and if abnormal, which contrast properties are harder to see. Depending on the frequency of the gratings that are harder to see, different types of eye disease or abnormality can be entertained; however, this is a very inexact way to differentiate ocular disease as there is significant overlap

## What the Patient Needs to Know

- This test checks your ability to distinguish between various contrasts or shades of objects.
- Each eye will be tested separately.
- Please wear your glasses for this test.
- Everyone has difficulty identifying the very dimmest objects. You need to guess when the objects are very dim.

between poor contrast sensitivity and various ocular abnormalities. This type of contrast sensitivity test has become the standard for documenting contrast vision, and will be described in detail in the next section.

## Contrast Sensitivity Function

Contrast sensitivity tests consisting of varying sinusoidal gratings can be used to obtain a contrast sensitivity function. These tests are similar to one another in design and generally consist of numerous circles containing sinusoidal gratings of various contrasts and frequencies. The contrast of the gratings ranges from 50% to 0.3% contrast or 30% to 0.3% contrast, depending on the manufacturer. The gratings are tilted at a specific angle, either to the right or left, or straight up and down. The top row of the chart has a grating with wide sinusoidal "bars." The widths of the bars are based on cycles per degree; the cycles per degree are referred to as spatial frequencies. Low frequency gratings have very few bars within the circle, while high frequency gratings have numerous bars within the circle (see Figure 2-31). The top row, known as row "A" on the chart, is a low frequency row with 1.5 cycles per degree (c/d). Row "B" has 3 c/d, row "C" has 6 c/d, row "D" has 12 c/d, and row "E" has 18 c/d. Each row follows the same contrast pattern ranging from the most contrast on the left-hand side to the least contrast on the right-hand side. The angle and width of the gratings, as well as the specific contrast, has been developed in the laboratory.

The tests generally use sinusoidal gratings that are of large, intermediate, and small widths; the aggregate of responses is called a contrast sensitivity function. When plotted on a graph, the results are known as a contrast sensitivity curve. The contrast sensitivity function is based on the premise that some things are visible, while others are not. Those gratings that are of very low contrast become invisible to the human eye at a level right below the individual's visual threshold. Also, the number of bars a person is able to see in a fixed space is dependent on visual resolution. There is a point when the bars (white next to dark) no longer appear as bars, but appear rather as solid gray. The last point where the bars are visible is known as a visual threshold.

The very low frequency gratings (1.5 c/d) and the very high frequency gratings (18 c/d) are more difficult to see by the normal eye than are those gratings of intermediate frequencies. This means that individuals will need more contrast to see the low and high frequency gratings, and less contrast to see the mid-range frequency gratings. A normal contrast sensitivity function obtained from this type of test will be lower at both the low and high frequency ends and higher in the middle as seen in Figure 2-32. When plotted, the contrast sensitivity function results in a contrast sensitivity curve that can be used to determine if the individual has normal contrast vision, and if not, what contrast and frequency properties results in a decreased visual threshold. An abnormality may be across the entire contrast sensitivity curve (Figure 2-33) or at specific fre-

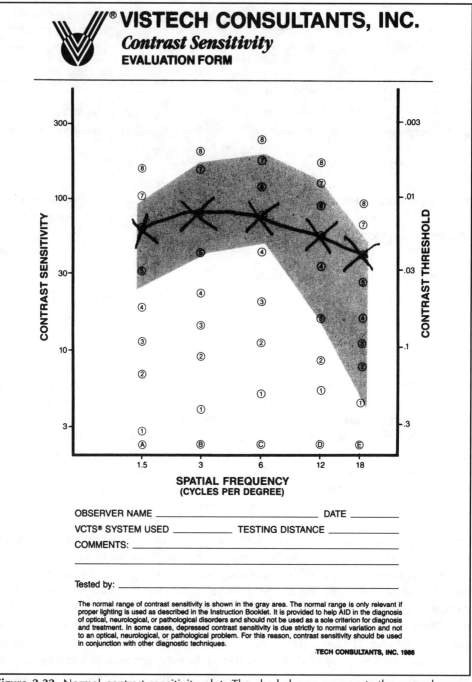

**Figure 2-32.** Normal contrast sensitivity plot. The shaded area represents the normal range. Everything below the shaded area suggests poor and abnormal contrast vision, whereas everything above the gray area suggests superior and supernormal contrast vision. (Reprinted with permission from Benes SC, McKinney K, Sanders LC, Miller M, Moberg M. *Advanced Ophthalmic Diagnostics and Therapeutics.* Thorofare, NJ: SLACK Incorporated; 1990.)

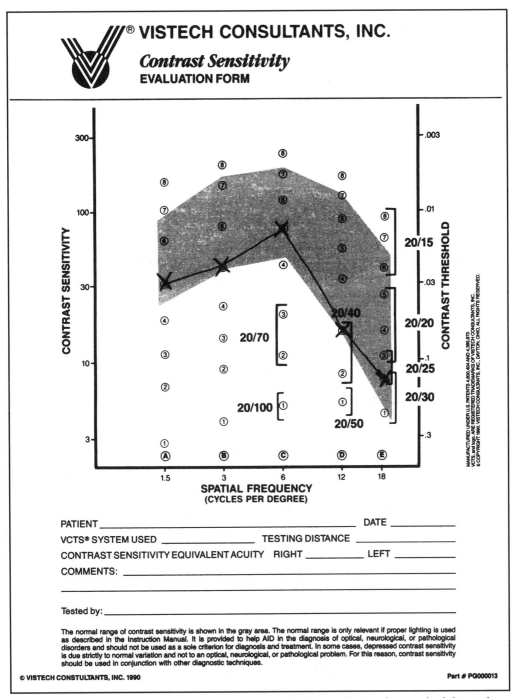

**Figure 2-33.** Contrast sensitivity plot that is within the lower limits of normal. If this is from an elderly individual it would be considered normal; however, if it were from a young patient it would be considered abnormal.

quencies (Figure 2-34). Some individuals may actually have better contrast sensitivity than most normal individuals, but this is not considered an abnormality even though it is outside the range of normal depicted on the chart (Figure 2-35).

The tests generally come on large rectangular charts (some are opaque, while others are back-illuminated) that are framed for easy installation on the wall (Figure 2-36). The opaque charts are made of special paper that will not fade if properly cared for. All of the charts have a grayish-white background that reduces the "ghost image" that can be produced by the barely-visible gratings if they are on white backgrounds. This ghost image might cue the patient into seeing gratings that otherwise would not be visible. The tests come with instruction manuals, score cards, several charts (to reduce the likelihood of memorization), and a light meter.

### Obtaining a Contrast Sensitivity Function

As with all contrast sensitivity tests, the patient should be seated at the proper distance wearing his or her spectacle correction. The patient should be shown the four practice circles on the bottom of the chart. One circle has gratings oriented toward the right, one toward the left, one up and down, and one is blank. This allows the patient to know what to look for, and that some circles will appear blank. This should eliminate any anxiety that the patient might have about seeing a blank circle.

Cover the worse eye with an occluder and ask the patient to start with row "A" on the left-hand side. Have the patient read across until the circle looks blank. The person should then go to row "B" and read from left to right until the circle is blank. This procedure should be repeated until all of the rows have been read. The test is then repeated on the other eye.

Each circle on the chart is depicted on the score sheet (see Figure 2-32). The examiner should put an "X" on the score sheet that depicts the last correctly identified circle in that row. (Some score sheets actually show the direction of the gratings, while others just depict the grating with a number.) This should be repeated for each row. The examiner then connects the "X's" with a line, and then tests the other eye. The score for the second eye can be placed on the same or a separate score sheet. If the same sheet is used, the second eye should be charted in such a way as to not be confusing. (One eye can be depicted with a solid line and the other eye with a broken line, or two different colors can be used. A legend should be included on the chart for easy interpretation.) Recording the responses from the two eyes on the same score sheet provides a graphic representation of the differences that might exist in the contrast vision of each eye.

### Score Sheet—Plotting the Contrast Sensitivity Curve

The score sheets may look somewhat different from one another depending on the manufacturer and the number of different tests that can be scored using the same score sheet (eg, distance and near). There are some similarities among the sheets as well. Along the bottom of every score sheet are the letters A through E, which correspond to the rows on the chart. Above each letter are eight circles with numbers ranging from 1 (on the bottom) to 8 (on the top). These numbers represent the gratings on the chart, and refer to the circle on the far left (1) and to the circle on the far right (8) in the corresponding row. Also, along the bottom of the score sheet are the spatial frequencies in cycles per degree that correspond to the gratings. The numbers on the right-hand side represent contrast threshold, which is the ability to discern minimum differences in contrast of adjacent surfaces. (If multiplied by 100, the resultant number would be equivalent to the percentage of contrast in the sinusoidal gratings. The number 0.3 for the contrast thresh-

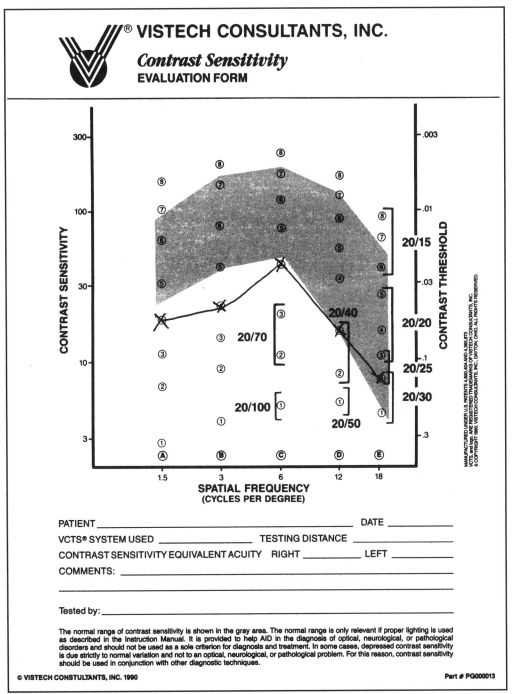

**Figure 2-34.** Abnormal contrast sensitivity plot from an elderly patient. The patient has great difficulty detecting lower frequency sinusoidal gratings.

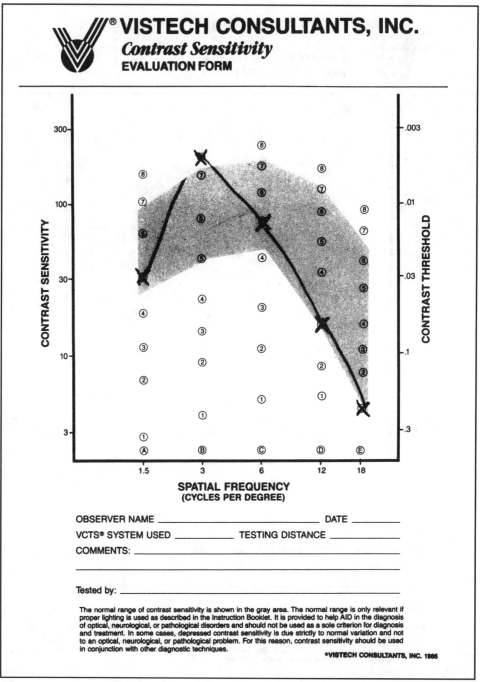

**Figure 2-35.** Contrast sensitivity plot showing above normal findings. This is a normal plot and suggests that the person's contrast sensitivity is actually better than normal. This would be comparable to someone having 20/10 visual acuity. (Reprinted with permission from Benes SC, McKinney K, Sanders LC, Miller M, Moberg M. *Advanced Ophthalmic Diagnostics and Therapeutics.* Thorofare, NJ: SLACK Incorporated; 1990.)

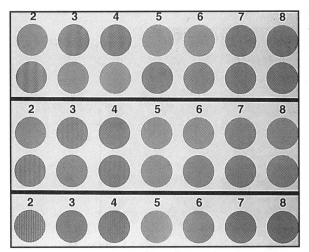

**Figure 2-36.** A back-illuminated contrast sensitivity chart. (Photograph by Nilo Davila.)

old means that the gratings are at 30% contrast.) The far right side of the score sheet has either a percentage of contrast number or a contrast threshold, depending on the manufacturer. The numbers on the right-hand side range from the most contrast that appears on the chart (at the bottom) to the least contrast that appears on the chart (at the top). The numbers on the left-hand side of the score sheet are the reciprocal of the contrast threshold, and are a numeric representation of the person's actual contrast vision as indicated per row. The numbers on the left-hand column range from the worst (at the bottom) to best (at the top), suggesting that the more circles that are correctly identified, the better the contrast vision. Individuals who score in the top part of the card (7s and 8s) have normal or super-normal contrast vision, and can see differences in adjacent surface luminance to the level of 0.3% contrast.

If score cards are used from a different contrast sensitivity test, it is important that the gratings are comparable between the two tests. Some charts start with a 50% contrast sinusoidal grating, while others start with a 30% contrast sinusoidal grating. This can be determined by looking at the right-hand legend of the score sheet. It is best to use only the manufacturer's score cards when documenting patient results.

## Test Results of the Contrast Sensitivity Curve

Each score sheet has a gray shaded area that represents the normal range of contrast sensitivity function for a general population (see Figure 2-32). However, evaluation of the score should not be based solely on whether or not the patient's score is within the normal range. For example, a young adult of age 20 should be able to see gratings that are not visible to an adult of age 70. Therefore, if a 20-year-old is just within the lower limits of normal, the test can be interpreted as abnormal (see Figure 2-33). If a person has a response that is above the gray shaded area, that would not constitute an abnormal test, but a super-normal test. The results suggest that the person's contrast vision is outside of the normal range because it is significantly better than normal (see Figure 2-35).

Contrast sensitivity function of the two eyes should be similar. If one eye has a contrast sensitivity curve that does not follow that of the other eye, the eye with the worse contrast sensitivity curve is probably abnormal. This would hold true even if the curve was within the normal range for the worse eye. Figure 2-37 represents similar contrast sensitivity curves, whereas Figure 2-38 shows

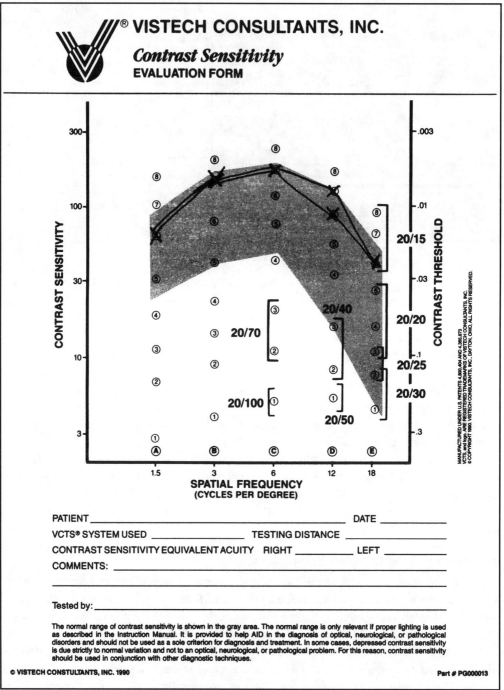

**Figure 2-37.** Contrast sensitivity plot showing that both eyes are normal and symmetric in function.

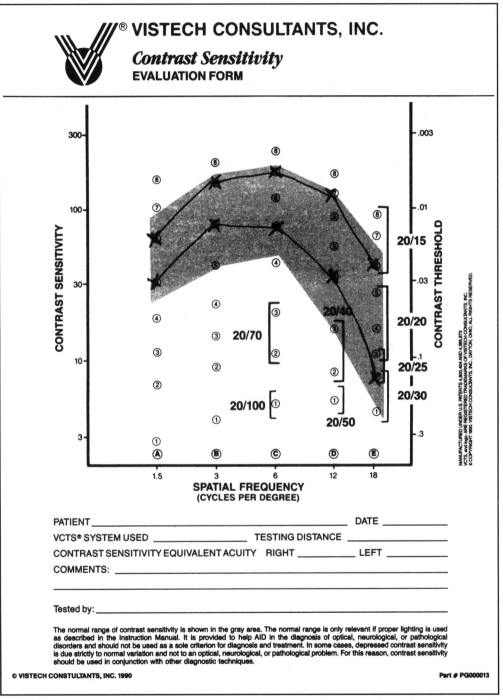

**Figure 2-38.** Contrast sensitivity plot showing asymmetric function. The right eye is clearly within the normal range, but the response from the left eye reveals poorer contrast vision (lower contrast sensitivity curve). This would be consistent with mild amblyopia, OS.

two curves that are significantly different from one another. This difference between the two eyes can be accounted for by the fact that the worse eye is amblyopic and has a Snellen acuity of 20/70.

Certain spatial frequencies are implicated in certain ocular diseases. Diseases of the brain often result in reduced contrast thresholds in the lower spatial frequencies. Diseases of the optic nerve (such as optic atrophy, glaucoma, and optic neuritis) often result in reduced contrast thresholds in the mid-range of spatial frequencies. Diseases of the macula and abnormalities and anomalies of the cornea and lens (such as cataract, keratoconus, and refractive error) result in reduced contrast thresholds in the higher spatial frequencies. These various conditions and their associated reductions in contrast thresholds have been established over the last several decades in both laboratory and clinical settings. However, there is significant overlap between frequency losses and ocular diseases, making it impossible to accurately associate frequency loss and ocular disease.

## Clinical Usefulness of Contrast Sensitivity Testing

Contrast sensitivity testing can be used to help determine the location of an abnormality, such as macular versus optic nerve disorders. However, such differentiation will often be done without the use of contrast sensitivity testing. Contrast sensitivity testing should generally be evaluated over multiple visits, just as one would perform Snellen acuity testing. Serial testing should give the examiner additional information about how a person is able to see and function over a period of time.

If a person has significant optic nerve disease while retaining relatively good central acuity (as in some optic neuritis cases), the contrast sensitivity results will be much more useful. Bilateral disease that is progressing in an asymmetric manner can also be better evaluated using contrast sensitivity testing. Functional assessment in preoperative cases, such as patients with cataracts or keratoconus, can be useful for justifying surgical intervention based on reduced contrast sensitivity function in the presence of relatively good visual acuity. Patients who are having difficulty with their contact lenses can be followed with contrast sensitivity testing, as improved contrast threshold suggests better contact lens fitting. Also, individuals with off-axis cylinder in their prescription can have their prescription refined by using the high frequency gratings as visual targets during refinement. (Better refinement results in better identification of high frequency gratings of low contrast.)

# Chapter 3

# Microbiology

## KEY POINTS

- Microbiology is the study of extremely small subcellular, single-celled, or multi-celled organisms.

- Microorganisms are everywhere in the environment, and some can cause eye disease.

- Proper identification of infectious ocular microorganisms is important in determining a more appropriate treatment of disease.

# Overview

Microbiology is the study of extremely small organisms that can only be viewed by means of standard or electron microscopy. These organisms may be single-celled, such as bacteria, or sub-cellular, such as viruses. These organisms are virtually everywhere, and are too numerous to count.

Although many of us are disdainful of these tiny organisms, their absence would have profoundly negative effects on humans. Many microorganisms remove unwanted waste from our environment. If microorganisms were to be completely eliminated from the face of the earth, we would be swimming in our own waste within several weeks. This would result in the demise of all mammals, including humans. Many of these microorganisms live naturally on our skin, in our intestines, and on our eyelashes. They help to keep us clean and digest our food. So, although we may not like the thought of these organisms being present virtually everywhere in our environment, they do serve an important purpose.

Unfortunately, we must take the good with the bad, and some of these microorganisms can make us very sick. When a new or unfamiliar microorganism enters the body, the individual will frequently become ill. The unfamiliar microorganism is referred to as a *foreign antigen,* which designates this organism as one against which the body raises an *immune response*. The body will not raise an immune response to a microorganism it is familiar with, such as the microorganisms that naturally occur in the human intestine. However, if an individual is exposed to a bacteria that is unfamiliar (or if a familiar bacteria migrates to an unusual place), illness may result.

When the body realizes that a bacterial foreign antigen is present, it will respond by trying to destroy the antigen. (The inflammation present at a wound site is the result of the body's immune response destroying the foreign antigen.) In many instances, the body's immune response will destroy the antigen efficiently; however, under other circumstances, assistance (by means of antibiotics, for example) will become necessary. A doctor may prescribe an antibiotic to assist in destroying the foreign bacteria, but this is not done because the immune system cannot do it on its own. Instead, the purpose is to eliminate the possibility of complications resulting from the inflammatory process. Scarring is an example.

An immune response is a natural occurrence within the body that results in the body's ability to fight off infection. In essence, it is a survival mechanism that the body possesses to use against microorganisms. Just as we would use weapons to fight off an invading army, the body uses the immune system to fight off invading microorganisms.

The immune response is generated by the immune system, which is part of the blood. There are two types of cells in the blood stream: the red blood cells and the white blood cells. The white blood cells (with one exception) make up the immune system. An individual with few white blood cells will have a poorly functioning immune system (as is the case with AIDS). Conversely, a person with a very high white blood cell count probably has an active infection that the body is fighting. The white blood cells destroy the foreign antigen, and will increase in number until virtually all of the invading organisms are destroyed. After that point, the immune system will return to normal, and the number of white blood cells present in the blood will go down to a normal range.

There are several types of white blood cells that make up the immune system. Depending on the type of foreign antigen present, the body will use more of one type of white blood cell than another type to fight the invading antigen. By understanding which white blood cell is associated with which type of antigen, a microbiologist may be able to determine the underlying cause of the immune response. (Namely, what type of foreign antigen is present and causing the problem.) A more detailed description of the immune system and the immune response will be given later.

Although most individuals have normally functioning immune systems and an efficient way to fight off infection, the best defense against infection is prevention. Within the healthcare setting, optometric and ophthalmic medical assistants want to eliminate patients' exposure to foreign antigens. We reduce or eliminate the possibility of exposure between patients by following "Universal Precautions" within our offices. Universal precautions are guidelines that have been developed over the years to reduce the risk of exposure to blood and bodily fluids that may contain foreign antigens (known as bloodborne pathogens). These precautions were established as a way to reduce the risk of exposure to fatal or very harmful diseases such as human immunodeficiency virus (HIV) or hepatitis B virus (HBV). However, certain guidelines also effectively reduce the risk of exposure to less serious diseases, such as epidemic keratoconjunctivitis (EKC). By following these guidelines within the clinical practice, we virtually eliminate the possibility of inadvertently exposing any patient, doctor, or ourselves to blood or bodily fluids. The American Academy of Ophthalmology (AAO) has designed specific guidelines for ophthalmic practices. A discussion of microbiology would not be complete without this information, which will be presented in Appendix B.

# Ocular Microbiology

As you are aware, a human being is constantly exposed to microorganisms. As a result, the eye is also exposed. These microorganisms include viruses, bacteria, fungi, protozoa, chlamydia, and (infrequently) multi-cellular parasites such as onchocerciasis (Table 3-1). Although these microorganisms are ubiquitous in the environment, the eye is generally not affected by these organisms. This is because a healthy, intact corneal epithelium is not very susceptible to invading antigens. It is not until the epithelium is disrupted that an infection generally occurs. The epithelium may be disrupted by such things as wearing of contact lenses too often or other types of trauma, exposure (due to lid anomalies), poor blinking, or poor tear production. Additionally, individuals who are susceptible to infection in general may also be susceptible to eye infections. Such individuals may have poor immune systems due to diseases such as HIV, or they may have been treated with chemotherapy to combat disorders such as cancer. The eyes of such patients may be more susceptible to bacterial, viral, fungal, chlamydial, or other infections. Moreover, a person with a previous herpes simplex viral infection who is exposed to yet another virus may develop a secondary herpes infection that may involve the eye.

Exposure to foreign antigens that affect the eye may result in typical symptoms such as pain, itching, tearing, discharge, and photophobia. However, the treatment for each antigen may be quite different. Differentiation of microorganisms can be done in several ways. First, the clinical appearance of the patient may lead to a diagnosis. Second, smears from the conjunctiva or cornea that are mounted on slides and viewed under the microscope may reveal the underlying cause of infection. Third, a scraping that is cultured on a particular medium and allowed to grow may reveal the offending antigen as well as which drugs might be effective in combating the antigen. Fourth, determining the location of the infection may help reveal the underlying antigen. Finally, viewing the other cells (immune cells) present in the smear may assist in determining the diagnosis.

## Viruses

Viruses are sub-cellular parasites that contain genetic material and have an outer protein coat (for protection). Because the virus is subcellular, it must have a host cell in order to reproduce

Table 3-1.
## Disease-Causing Antigens of the Eye

| Viruses | Bacteria | Fungi | Chlamydia | Protozoa | Multi-Celled Parasites |
|---------|----------|-------|-----------|----------|------------------------|
| Herpes simplex | *Cocci* | Candida | Inclusion | Acanthamoeba | *Nematodes* |
| Herpes zoster | Gram-positive | Fusarium | conjunctivitis | Toxoplasmosis | Toxocariasis |
| Adenovirus | Staphlycoccus | Aspergillus | Trachoma | Pneumocytosis | Onchocerciasis |
| | Streptococcus | | | | Loiasis |
| | | | | | (Loa loa worm) |
| | Gram-negative | | | | Trichinosis |
| | Gonococcus | | | | Ancylostoma |
| | (Neisseria gonorrhoeae) | | | | canimun |
| | Meningococcus | | | | (possible cause |
| | (Neisseria meningitidis) | | | | of DUSN) |
| | Neisseria catarrhalis | | | | |
| | | | | | *Cestodes* |
| | *Bacilli* | | | | Cysticercosis |
| | Gram-positive | | | | |
| | Corynebacterium | | | | *Trematodes* |
| | Bacillus | | | | Schistosomiasis |
| | Mycobacterium | | | | Seen primarily |
| | | | | | in developing |
| | Gram-negative | | | | countries. |
| | Pseudomonas | | | | |
| | Haemophilus | | | | |
| | Moraxella | | | | |
| | | | | | |
| | *Spirilla* | | | | |
| | Treponema pallidum | | | | |
| | (spirochette that causes syphilis) | | | | |

DUSN = diffuse unilateral subacute neuroretinitis

itself. The virus infects a naturally-occurring cell within a person (that acts as a host for the virus) and mixes its genetic material with that of the infected cell's genetic material. The infected cell (which is now the cellular host for the virus) then behaves like the virus and produces new viruses within itself. The host cell is either destroyed by the virus (the cell more or less bursts open, referred to as cell lysis) or it acts as an incubator for the virus and constantly produces new viral material (no lysis is involved in this case). This infection of the healthy cell(s) and subsequent viral production is what makes us sick.

When the immune system realizes that the host cell contains foreign genetic material, the immune system raises a response against that contaminated cell, and subsequently destroys the virus. The process of destroying virus-infected cells takes about 10 days to complete. That is why a person is sick with a viral infection for approximately 10 days. However, the individual may have been exposed to the virus weeks before showing any symptoms of illness.

Viruses are not destroyed by antibiotics. Neither have scientists been able to destroy infected host cells without killing uninfected, healthy cells of the same organ or region of the body. Many anti-viral medications act in various ways to reduce the virus's ability to mix its genetic material with that of the host cell's. In some rare instances antibiotics are prescribed to individuals with viral infections, but this is to reduce the possibility of secondary bacterial infections and not as a means to control the virus itself.

After exposure to a particular virus the body generally will become immune to that virus, meaning that an efficient immune response is immediately activated on the next exposure to the virus and the person will not get sick. This is the principle behind vaccinations, where dead or weakened viruses are introduced to the body so that an immune response can be raised with little possibility of the person becoming seriously ill. The next time the person is exposed to that same virus the immune response (triggered into action by immunologic memory) will be guaranteed, and the person will not become sick. Immunologic memory is not perfect, however, so individuals must receive booster vaccines in order to keep the immunologic response efficient.

Many viruses, such as polio and smallpox, have been controlled through vaccination. Other viruses are not effectively controlled by vaccination. Generally, those not controlled through vaccination are retroviruses, which contain RNA genetic material instead of DNA. Retroviruses frequently lay dormant in a host cell and become reactivated when the person is under stress or exposed to other viruses. A common retrovirus is the herpes simplex virus.

There are three viruses that are generally associated with eye conditions— the herpes simplex virus, the herpes zoster virus, and the adenovirus.

The most common ocular herpetic manifestation is herpes simplex dendritic keratitis, which results in a corneal lesion (Figure 3-1). Because herpes simplex also causes the common cold sore, a lip lesion is frequently found in those with an active herpetic corneal ulcer. This corneal lesion has a very typical dendritic (branched) pattern best seen when stained with fluorescein. A recurrent corneal lesion may result in permanent scarring. In this case a corneal transplant may be required for improvement of visual acuity. In some instances the new graft will become re-infected with the herpetic virus. Herpes can also manifest in areas around the eye including the lids and lid margins. Infections in this area rarely result in reduced visual acuity. In very rare instances herpes can cause an infection of the brain known as encephalitis, which can result in the severe reduction of vision if the visual cortex is involved.

Herpes zoster is caused by the same virus that causes shingles and chickenpox. Both herpes zoster and shingles generally occur in older adults or individuals who have compromised immune systems (such as individuals with an HIV infection). The zoster infection generally occurs along the 5th cranial nerve and will not cross the mid-line of the face. The individual may experience facial pain before the lesions appear. The lesions, which usually appear on the forehead and eyelids, generally erupt and result in scabs that may leave permanent scars on the face (Figure 3-2). The eyelids are edematous and there is often tearing. If the lesions on the face involve the tip of the nose, there will be corneal involvement as well. The cornea may have fine white subepithelial opacities or fine dendritic opacities. Ocular complications may include glaucoma, iritis, scleritis, or persistent corneal opacities.

The adenoviruses cause several ocular conditions including epidemic keratoconjunctivitis (EKC). The infection results in a fairly painful ocular condition that generally occurs bilaterally because it is so easily spread. Initially, the individual notes moderate pain, redness, and tearing. This is followed by significant photophobia, lid edema, chemosis, conjunctival hyperemia, and epithelial keratitis. This condition lasts about 3 weeks, but on occasion will last somewhat longer. As EKC is very contagious, it can be a cause of real concern within the eyecare practice. Frequently the virus is spread through contaminated eye droppers. The contamination occurs when the conjunctiva or eyelashes of an infected patient makes contact with the eye dropper. The solution then contains the virus that will be used on the next unsuspecting person if the eye dropper is not discarded. Spread of EKC can occur through direct contact between the eyecare professional and the infected patient, with subsequent contact with a non-infected individual. Inade-

**Figure 3-1.** Recurrent herpes simplex dendritic keratitis. (Reprinted with permission of the American Academy of Ophthalmology. *External Disease and Cornea: A Slide-Script Program.* 2nd ed. San Francisco, Calif: The American Academy of Ophthalmology; 1988.)

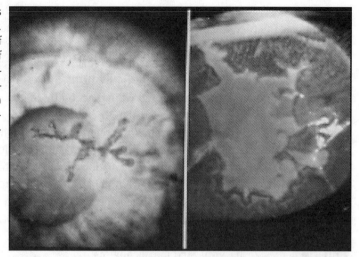

**Figure 3-2.** A patient with herpes zoster. (Reprinted with permission from Stein HA, Slatt BJ, Stein RM, *The Ophthalmic Assistant.* St. Louis, Mo. CV Mosby Co, 1988.)

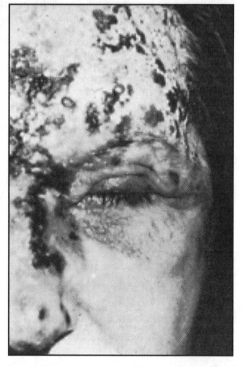

quate hand washing has been reported as the cause of one EKC epidemic.[1] Care must be taken to insure that adequate hand washing (as well as other precautions) occurs between patient contacts (see Appendix B).

## Bacteria

Bacteria are single cell organisms. These simple organisms contain all of the material necessary for energy production and cell reproduction. Bacteria reproduce asexually by means of cell division (called *simple fission*). When the bacterium splits, it produces two identical bacteria, referred to as "daughters." This splitting can be extremely fast, and under good conditions one bacterium can result in over 16 million new bacteria within one day. Bacteria generally live in soft tissue, blood, and bone. As the bacteria consume these tissues, they produce a toxic waste. The waste from the bacteria, along with the destruction of the tissue, is what makes people sick.

Bacteria are classified by means of their shape—round, rod-shaped, or spiral. Round, spherical bacteria are called "cocci". A single spherical bacterium is called a coccus. Generally, cocci grow in chains, clusters, or pairs (Figure 3-3). *Pneumococcus* grows in pairs, *Staphylococcus* grows in grape-like clusters, whereas *Streptococcus* grows in a chain, like a string of pearls. Any bacteria name that ends in "coccus" designates it as a round, spherical bacteria.

Rod-shaped bacteria are called "bacilli;" a single bacterium is called a bacillus. They grow in chains or singularly. Although they are essentially rod-shaped, they can be short, long, thin, rounded, straight, or slightly curved (Figure 3-4). Again, bacilli can be identified by their appearance. *Pseudomonas* and *Mycobacterium* are both rod-shaped bacteria that cause ocular infections. *Pseudomonas* is a very aggressive organism which can cause great and rapid devastation to the eye. This bacteria is often the cause of corneal ulcers in contact lens wearers.

Bacteria that are both rod-shaped and spiral-shaped are called "spirilla." These are very small bacteria which cannot be seen easily under a standard microscope. Special techniques must be employed in order to see spirilla bacteria. Frequently cultures must be obtained, and the culture patterns must be observed in order to classify this bacteria. The type of spirilla bacteria which causes syphilis is called a spirochete (Figure 3-5).

## Fungi

Fungi are a group of simple plants that do not possess chlorophyll (green color found in most plants). They occur virtually everywhere in the environment. Many fungi can be seen by the unaided eye and can include large multi-cellular plants such as mushrooms. Others must be viewed under the microscope or in a culture, such as single-cell yeast fungi. Microscopic fungi are generally larger than bacteria. Since fungi do not possess chlorophyll, a necessary ingredient for photosynthesis and food production for plants, fungi must live off of a host in order to survive. Frequently, fungi are found on other plants which act as host plants. Fungi reproduce by spore production. They do not generally affect the eye; however if an ocular fungal infection is suspected, the person usually has a history of exposure to some type of plant material. (The person may report having been scratched in the eye by a tree branch, for example.) Microscopic fungi that affect the eye generally grow in interlacing filaments or in a rounded form. The fungi most commonly reported in ophthalmic cases are *Candida, Fusarium,* and *Aspergillus.*

## *Chlamydia*

*Chlamydia* is an unusual organism because it behaves in ways that are reminiscent of both viruses and bacteria. In the past it was actually classified as a "large virus," but more recently it has been found to be a gram-negative bacteria. (The terms gram-negative and gram-positive refer to a staining technique, and will be explained later.) Unlike most bacteria, chlamydia needs a host cell for reproduction. This is very similar to the reproductive cycle of viruses. The organism attaches to a host cell which subsequently surrounds the chlamydia. The *Chlamydia* goes on to form a cytoplasmic inclusion body within which cell division takes place, ultimately resulting in numerous infectious cells. The chlamydia cells within the host cell undergo simple fission just as bacteria do. After extensive cell fission, the host cell ruptures and the new chlamydia cells are released to infect other potential host cells.

**Figure 3-3.** Gram-positive streptococcus and white blood cells. Note the round shape of the bacterium. (Photograph courtesy of Melvin Trousdale, PhD.)

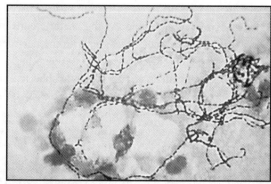

**Figure 3-4.** Gram-positive bacillus bacteria. Note the rod-like shape of the bacterium. (Photograph courtesy of Melvin Trousdale, PhD.)

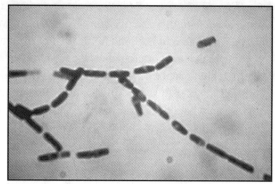

**Figure 3-5.** Spirochete. (Photograph courtesy of Melvin Trousdale, PhD.)

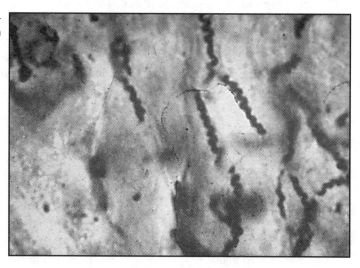

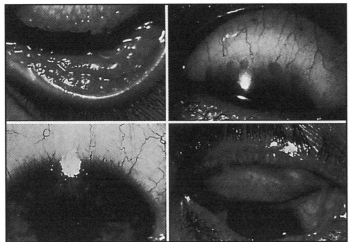

**Figure 3-6.** Trachoma infection of the eye. (Reprinted with permission of the American Academy of Ophthalmology. *External Disease and Cornea: A Slide-Script Program.* 2nd ed. San Francisco, Calif: The American Academy of Ophthalmology; 1988.)

Trachoma is the most common chlamydial ocular infection (Figure 3-6). It is very infectious and one of the leading causes of blindness worldwide. It is not common within most developed countries. Trachoma affects the conjunctiva and the corneal epithelium, resulting in serious corneal scarring that leads to blindness. A second chlamydial infection, involving mostly newborns, is caused by venereal chlamydia. It is also very infectious and looks histopathologically similar to the chlamydia that causes trachoma.

## Protozoa

Protozoa are one-celled animals, some of which can infect the eye. Amoeba (also spelled ameba) are the simplest of the protozoa. The amoeba measures about 0.01 of an inch in length and lives in water, moist soil, and the bodies of some animals and humans. Most amoebas are harmless to humans, but one type causes severe dysentery. Amoebas generally live on other microscopic organisms such as bacteria. Amoebas reproduce by means of cell fission, which produces two new amoebas that are identical to one another.

In recent years amoebic infection of the cornea has become more common. The specific organism involved, *Acanthamoeba*, can be found in numerous locations including water, hot tubs, and soil. In the past, many soft contact lens wearers used homemade saline solution made with saline tablets and unsterile tap water that may have contained *Acanthamoeba*. As a result, certain wearers became infected with this organism. Some soft contact lens wearers who spend time in hot tubs while wearing their lenses can also become infected. There has been a concerted effort to eliminate corneal Acanthamoeba infection. Individuals who make their own saline are advised to use sterile water. Also, soft contact lens wearers have been advised not to wear the lenses in certain environments such as hot tubs.

Acanthamoeba infection can be extremely damaging to the cornea (Figure 3-7). Despite vigorous medical intervention, many individuals with corneal Acanthamoeba infection must undergo corneal transplantation, with about one-third of the grafts becoming reinfected.

Another protozoa that affects the eye is toxoplasmosis. The protozoa is usually ingested or absorbed by a pregnant woman who transmits it to her developing offspring. The protozoa gets lodged in the eye and causes permanent damage, generally to the retina and choroid. Active toxoplasmosis will result in vitreous haze and severely reduced visual acuity. After an active infection,

**Figure 3-7.** Electron microscope picture of *Acanthamoeba* on a cornea. (Photograph courtesy of Melvin Trousdale, PhD.)

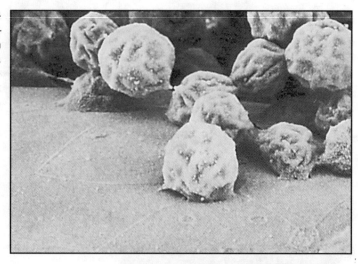

**Figure 3-8.** Chorioretinal scar from a toxoplasmosis infection. (Reprinted with permission from Stein HA, Slatt BJ, Stein RM. *The Ophthalmic Assistant.* St. Louis, Mo: CV Mosby Co; 1988.)

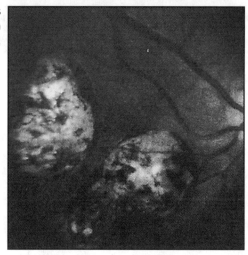

a scar will remain in the area of the lesion. If this scar is near the macula, vision may be affected (Figure 3-8).

## Multi-Celled Parasites

Infection of the eye by multi-celled parasitic microorganisms is more common in underdeveloped countries. These diseases include onchocerciasis (the cause of river blindness), Loa loa eye worm, and intraretinal worms (causing diffuse unilateral subacute neuroretinitis, or DUSN). Most of these disorders are distinguishable by examining the patient with a slit lamp or with an ophthalmoscope. In some situations visualization is not possible, and biopsies of the involved tissues must be taken.

## Identification of the Infectious Antigen

Although many of the organisms just described result in similar-looking anterior segment disorders, the underlying infectious agents respond differently to various treatments. While it is important to properly identify the causative organism, prompt treatment is also essential. It is therefore unlikely that a physician will wait for a definitive diagnosis, but will rather start treatment immediately. Diagnosis will be based on patient complaints and ocular findings. Once the foreign antigen is isolated, treatment strategy will be modified to best combat the infectious process.

As suggested earlier, many antigens are difficult to see with the unaided eye. In such instances several things can be done to assist in identification. Smears and scrapings can be taken for mounts or cultures. Inflammatory cells from the host may be identified on mounts as well, assisting in an indirect identification of the organism. Finally, biopsies can be taken of the involved tissues when identification is impossible by other means.

A smear or culture should be considered in any eye with an acute or chronic conjunctivitis of unknown etiology, or in any conjunctivitis in a newborn. Any eye with a corneal ulcer should also be·cultured. In some instances the adnexa of the eye will need to be cultured. Finally, eyes that have developed a postoperative infection will need to be cultured via a vitreal tap.

In many situations the assistant will be able to take a smear and make either a slide or a culture. Proper handling of specimens will result in more accurate antigen identification, which will ultimately result in appropriate therapeutic intervention for the patient.

## Obtaining the Organism for Staining or Culture

Smears can be taken from the infected tissue of the eye or from the ocular discharge. Collection can be done by gently scraping the affected area with either a cotton swab (for cultures) or a spatula (for staining) (Figures 3-9 and 3-10). If the affected area includes the cornea, the ophthalmologist must perform the scraping or swabbing because of the potential damage that could occur to the cornea if done improperly. The spatula or cotton swab is rubbed against the advancing area of infection to ensure that the offending antigen is obtained. Individuals are advised to wear protective gloves while doing scrapings or swabbings. If gloves are not worn, individuals must wash the hands thoroughly both before and after the procedure.

### Making a Stain

There are several types of stains that are frequently used within the ophthalmic practice. They include the Gram stain which is used to detect bacteria, the GMS stain which is used to detect fungi, and the Giemsa and Wright stains which are used to differentiate cell structure (usually blood cells of the immune system that help in antigen identification).

Making a stain is like following any set of written instructions. One must stick to the directions and not deviate from them or the organism will not be made visible. There are commercially available stain kits or you can purchase the necessary ingredients separately. The directions may be slightly different depending on which kit you buy, as not all kits contain the exact same items. The following are general directions for making each type of stain.

#### Gram Stain

The Gram stain is used to detect and classify bacteria. When making a Gram stain, one must start out by smearing the specimen evenly on a clean, dry glass microscope slide (Figure 3-11). The smear should be thinly spread to eliminate clumping of cells on the slide. The best way to identify cells is to see the whole cell. This can best be done if the microscope light adequately illuminates the whole cell. If there is a glob of cells on the slide then the light will not pass through individual cells, making cell identification difficult.

**Figure 3-9.** A moistened sterile cotton swab can be used to remove ocular material that is to be cultured. (Reprinted with permission from Stein HA, Slatt BJ, Stein RM. *The Ophthalmic Assistant.* St. Louis, Mo: CV Mosby Co; 1988.)

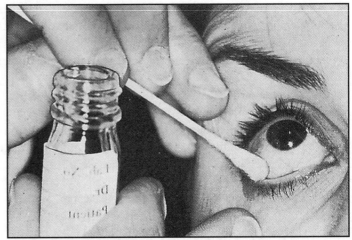

**Figure 3-10.** A moistened sterile spatula can be used to remove ocular material that is to be cultured. (Reprinted with permission from Stein HA, Slatt BJ, Stein RM. *The Ophthalmic Assistant.* St. Louis, Mo: CV Mosby Co; 1988.)

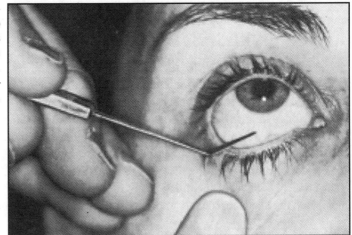

**Figure 3-11.** Specimen being smeared on a clean glass slide. (Reprinted with permission from Stein HA, Slatt BJ, Stein RM. *The Ophthalmic Assistant.* St. Louis, Mo: CV Mosby Co; 1988.)

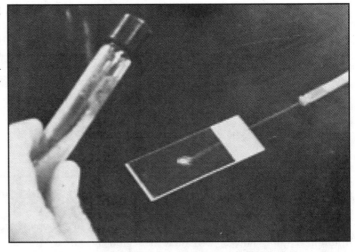

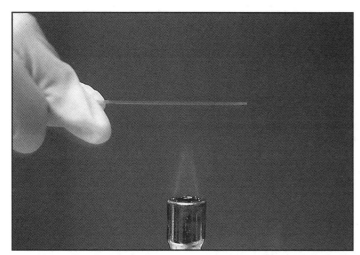

**Figure 3-12.** The smear is next fixed onto the slide by means of a Bunsen burner. A gelatin adhesive can be sprayed onto the slide prior to smearing the specimen onto the slide instead of using a Bunsen burner. (Photograph by Nilo Davila.)

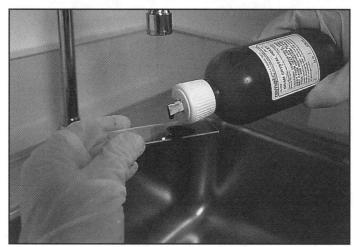

**Figure 3-13.** The smear is covered with a gentian violet solution for 1 minute and then rinsed in tap water. (Photograph by Nilo Davila.)

Next, the smear is fixed by means of a flame, usually a Bunsen burner (Figure 3-12). The slide is passed through the flame of the burner until the smear is dry. The smear is then covered with a gentian violet solution for 1 minute (Figure 3-13) then rinsed with gently running tap water. Next, the smear is covered with Gram's iodine for 1 minute (Figure 3-14). After 1 minute the slide is rinsed in running tap water, and then decolorized with 95% ethyl alcohol (or acetone) until the color no longer bleeds off the section (Figure 3-15). Decolorization may take about 20 seconds. The slide is next washed off with tap water and stained with 1% safranin for 3 minutes (Figure 3-16). The slide is once again washed with tap water, gently blotted, and allowed to air dry.

When observed under the microscope, gram-positive bacteria will stain dark blue and gram-negative bacteria will stain red. Gram-positive cocci bacteria include *Staphylococcus* and *Streptococcus*, while gram-negative cocci bacteria include *Gonococcus* and *Meningococcus*. Gram-positive bacilli bacteria include *Cornebacterium*, *Bacillus*, and *Mycobacterium*, while gram-negative bacilli bacteria include *Pseudomonas*, *Haemophilus*, and *Moraxella* (Table 3-2). Other cells or tissues will be stained pale yellow to pink.

**Figure 3-14.** Next, the smear is covered with Gram's iodine for 1 minute. (Photograph by Nilo Davila.)

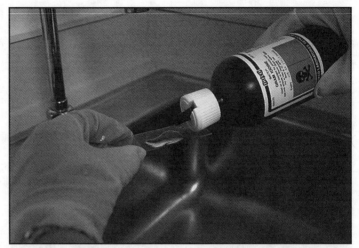

**Figure 3-15.** After 1 minute the slide is rinsed in running tap water and then decolorized with ethyl alcohol. (Photograph by Nilo Davila.)

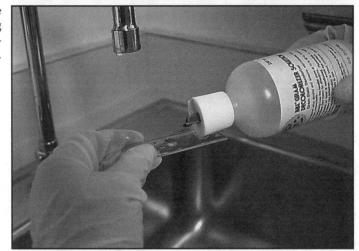

**Figure 3-16.** The slide is rinsed in tap water and stained with 1% safranin for 3 minutes, then rinsed again. The slide is gently blotted, allowed to air dry, and then is ready for viewing under a microscope. (Photograph by Nilo Davila.)

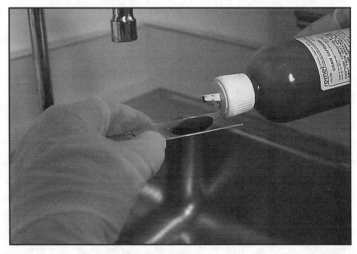

Table 3-2.
## Common Bacterial Ocular Infections

| Organism | Microscopic Form | Gram Stain | Culture Medium | Colonies in Culture | Pathology | Potential Findings |
|---|---|---|---|---|---|---|
| *Staphylococcus* | cocci in cluster, but may vary | + | any nutrient | opaque, round, smooth, raised, glistening, 1 to 2 mm diameter | pyogenic, necrotizing | blepharitis, hordeolum, conjunctivitis, keratitis, cellulitis |
| *Streptococcus* | cocci in chains | + | enriched (blood) | pinpoint, grayish, 2 to 4 mm zone where blood in medium has been digested | watery discharge, diffuse, spreads rapidly, often associated with injury | cellulitis |
| *S. pneumonia* (pneumonia) | lancet-shaped diplococci | + | blood agar | small, depressed in center, shiny, surrounded by zone of green | stringy discharge, invasive, edema sudden onset | hypopyon, keratitis, chronic dacrocystitis, conjunctivitis (acute) |
| *Neisseria gonorrhoeae* (VD) | paired kidney-shaped intra-cellular organism | – | chocolate or blood agar | clear, glistening, large irregular edges | purulent discharge, localized | ophthalmia neonatorum, conjunctivitis, marginal corneal ulcer |
| *Neisseria meningitidis* | small, paired | – | chocolate or blood agar | round, low, convex, glistening, gray or gray/blue tinge | petechial or purpuric skin rash | corneal ulcer |
| *Neisseria catarrhalis* | paired | – | chocolate or blood agar | white, smooth and opaque | normal throat species | conjunctivitis |
| *Corynebacterium* | slender rods in pairs or short chains | + | blood agar, Tinsdale agar | gray-black colonies with brown halo | purulent discharge | conjunctivitis |
| *Bacillus* | long rods in chains | + | blood agar | flat & irregular, 4 to 5 mm in diameter, may have undulate margin | associated with injury | endoph-thalmitis |
| *Mycobacterium* | typical rods | acid fast | egg, Lowenstein-Jensen | smooth/rough, pigmented or nonpigmented, (depends on species), generally slow-growing | immune cell infiltrate | conjunctivitis, corneal ulcer |

Table 3-2 continued.
## Common Bacterial Ocular Infections

| Organism | Microscopic Form | Gram Stain | Culture Medium | Colonies in Culture | Pathology | Potential Findings |
|---|---|---|---|---|---|---|
| *Pseudomonas* | single or pair, short chains or groups | – | blood agar or fluid medium | dark greenish-gray with zone of bluish-green, sweet hay-like odor | purulent destructive necrosis | severe hypopyon, keratitis, endoph-thalmitis, corneal abcess, cellulitis |
| *Haemophilus* | tiny slender rod, no particular arrangement | – | chocolate or blood agar | pinpoint, translucent, glistening | mucoid discharge | conjunctivitis (epidemic) |
| *Moraxella* | paired | – | enriched blood | small, pinpoint (less than 0.5 mm) | subacute or chronic catarrhal | conjunctivitis, endoph-thalmitis |
| *Treponema pallidum* (syphilis) | slender, curved, flagellated | not used | no *in vitro* growth | none | 3 stages | primary: chancres secondary: ulcerative blepharoco-njunctivis tertiary: gummas |

### GMS Stain

The GMS stain is used to detect *Pneumocystis carinii* (which causes a fatal pneumonia in AIDS patients) and fungi (including *Aspergillus* and *Candida*). This stain will likely be performed at a local laboratory and not a private ophthalmology office, because it is quite complicated. The following is a brief description on how to make this slide. Smears are air dried and are then placed in a Coplin jar containing 10% chromic acid for exactly 10 minutes. The chromic acid is then discarded and the slide is washed in tap water for a few seconds. Next, the slide is placed in 1% sodium metabisulfite for 1 minute; the sodium metabisulfite is then discarded and the slide is washed in hot tap water for 1 minute until the Coplin jar is hot. A freshly prepared solution of methenamine silver solution is poured into the Coplin jar onto the slide, where it remains until the smear becomes a golden brown (usually 2 minutes). The methenamine silver is discarded and the slide is rinsed in hot water that is gradually cooled so as not to crack the Coplin jar. The slide is removed from the jar and rinsed in distilled water. This is followed by a placing a small amount of 1% gold chloride on the slide for about 10 seconds. The slide is rinsed in distilled water, and then placed in a solution of 5% sodium thiosulfate solution for 3 minutes. The slide is again rinsed in distilled water and allowed to air dry. The fungi then can be viewed under the microscope and will have a brownish color.

### Giemsa Stain

The Giemsa stain is used to view cells from the immune system and other cells that may be present with the foreign antigen. (The immune system will be discussed in detail later in this chapter.) Start by smearing the specimen on a clean, dry slide. Let the specimen air dry. After it has dried completely, the slide is fixed with an absolute methyl alcohol solution for 5 minutes. Then the slide is placed in a Coplin jar over a sink, where it is flooded with working May-Grunwald stain and then left to stand in the stain for 6 minutes. The slide must be agitated in the solution every 30 seconds or so to assure proper staining. The mixture is poured off and the slide is washed in a phosphate buffer solution at 6.8 pH until no more color bleeds off. The slide is then placed in a working Giemsa stain for 13 minutes. The slide must be agitated in the solution to assure proper staining. The slide is again rinsed in a phosphate buffer until the slide no longer bleeds color, and is then allowed to stand in the phosphate solution for 3 minutes. The slide is then air dried and ready for viewing.

### Wright Stain

The Wright stain is used to view cells from the immune system as well as other cells that may be present with the foreign antigen. (The immune system will be discussed in detail later in this chapter.) In many instances the antigen itself is not visible (particularly true in cases of viral infection). In order to determine the type of infectious process present, the observation of the host's inflammatory cells will give the ophthalmologist a hint as to the underlying cause of the infection. The Wright stain is used to view these other cells.

First, carefully place the specimen on a clean and dry slide. Allow the specimen to air dry. Cover the entire specimen with a small amount of Wright stain (about 10 drops) and allow the stain to remain on the slide for 1 minute. After 1 minute, add the same amount of distilled water to the slide (about 10 drops) to create a stain and distilled water mixture. The water and stain solution should remain on the slide for an additional 10 minutes. At the end of 10 minutes, drain off the solution from the slide and rinse in distilled water until the slide no longer bleeds. Allow the slide to air dry.

## Making a Culture

Producing a culture for organism identification is very important in making an accurate diagnosis. For any culture, the organism is taken from the eye and placed in a petri dish or tube containing a specific medium (liquid or gel containing nutrients) to enhance organism growth. In most instances, the culture is done in a laboratory by individuals who specialize in microbiology. In other cases, the culture is actually made in the eye clinic. The latter is generally true if a hospital or other laboratory is very close. If no laboratory is close by, the specimen must be kept protected so that a culture can be made once the cotton swab containing the organism has been transported to the laboratory.

The sterile cotton swab is first moistened with either sterile saline or sterile glucose broth, then swabbed across the affected area of the eye (usually the conjunctiva of the lower fornix) several times to assure that the organism is on the cotton swab. If the specimen is going to be sent out to a laboratory that is not close, the cotton swab is placed in a glass vial containing Stuart's transport medium. If a laboratory is close by, the culture can be made in the clinic. The swab is gently streaked across the medium in the petri dish. In some instances letters are actually drawn in the medium (such as "RE" for right eye) using the swab (Figure 3-17).

The type of culture medium used is based on the type of organism that is suspected depending on clinical presentation. Blood and chocolate agar are used to culture bacteria. Thioglucollate broth is used to culture anaerobic bacteria, while Sabouraud's dextrose agar is used to culture fungi. Lowenstein-Jensen medium is used to culture the organisms causing both tuberculosis and leprosy, and the Thayer-Martin plate is used to culture gonococcus bacteria.

**Figure 3-17.** The cotton swab or spatula is gently streaked across the medium in the petri dish. (Reprinted with permission from Stein HA, Slatt BJ, Stein RM. *The Ophthalmic Assistant.* St. Louis, Mo: CV Mosby Co; 1988.)

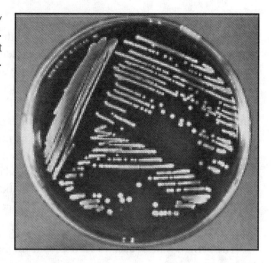

Once the organism has been swabbed across the petri dish, the dish is stored for 24 hours in an incubator set at 37° C. This allows time for bacterial growth. In the event that few organisms are then found, the dish should be incubated for a second 24 hour period. Fungi take a few weeks to grow and viruses (which are cultured on special medium) may take as long as 1 month to culture. In many instances it is actually easier to identify viruses through antibody tests of the blood than it is to culture the virus.

Another important aspect of culturing bacteria is to determine which antibiotic is most effective at killing the bacterial organism. This is called a sensitivity test. Disks containing different types of antibiotics (these are coded by numbers and/or colors) can be placed on a medium that has been smeared with bacteria. As the bacteria grow, they will avoid growing around disks that contain antibiotics to which the bacteria is sensitive. The antibiotic disk with the least bacterial growth around it will likely be chosen to treat the infected eye. (There may be several antibiotics that effectively kill the antigen; however, the antibiotic that should be used would be the most effective antibiotic, not just an effective antibiotic.)

In many instances when a patient comes into the clinic with a presumed bacterial infection, the ophthalmologist will prescribe a broad spectrum antibiotic that is known to kill many types of bacteria, and a slide of the organism will not be made. Instead, a sensitivity test will be performed and the ophthalmologist will then change to the antibiotic that is more effective at killing the bacteria (Figure 3-18).

# The Immune System

White blood cells and other fluids within the blood stream (primarily growth factors) provide us with a way to fight off infection. This is known as the immune system. The blood stream is made up of mostly red blood cells. However, if there is an infectious agent within the body, the body will activate an immune response which will increase the overall number of white blood cells present in the blood stream. In addition, there will be a higher concentration of the specific type of white blood cell necessary to fight the particular infection.

There are two general types of white blood cells that make up the immune system. The first type, called lymphocytes, respond to specific foreign antigens. The lymphocytes look for new foreign antigens that the individual has never before encountered, as well as specific antigens that the

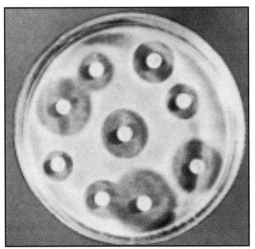

**Figure 3-18.** Sensitivity test to determine which antibiotic is most effective in killing the particular bacteria. The antibiotic saturated disk with the least bacterial growth around it would be considered the one containing the most effective antibiotic. (Reprinted with permission from Stein HA, Slatt BJ, Stein RM. *The Ophthalmic Assistant*. St. Louis, Mo: CV Mosby Co; 1988.)

individual has encountered previously. There are two types of lymphocytes, the T-cell lymphocyte and the B-cell lymphocyte. The T-cell lymphocyte changes its outer protein coat by means of DNA rearrangement so that when a foreign antigen is encountered for the first time, the immune system will be able to raise a response. The B-cell lymphocyte changes the DNA of its antibody receptor sites so that foreign antigens will attach to it. When a foreign antigen attaches itself to the cell surface of either a B-cell or T-cell lymphocyte, replication of that particular lymphocyte with that antigen-specific surface will occur rapidly. B-cell lymphocyte activation and reproduction results in the release of antibodies. The antibodies signal to other white blood cells that a foreign antigen is present and that it is time to go to work. The T-cell lymphocyte activation results in massive replication of that type of T-cell. The T-cells directly destroy the foreign antigen.

In some instances, the newly-encountered infectious agent is so devastating to the body that the immune system cannot fight it off in time to survive (as was true when Cortez came to the New World and brought smallpox to the indigenous populations). However, under most circumstances, the immune system will work efficiently against newly encountered foreign antigens.

Viruses, and to a lesser extent other foreign antigens, change their outer protein coats as a means of survival. By slight changes of its coat, the virus is able to out-maneuver the human immune system for several days. (It takes the immune system about 10 days to raise an immune response to this "new" virus.) The next encounter with the same virus will result in a full attack by the immune system and the individual will not become ill. If a new virus is encountered that is similar to one that the person has already encountered, the immune system will raise a response more quickly, thus reducing the amount of time the individual is sick. If the virus is a completely new strain, then the immune system will have to "start from scratch" in raising an immune response, resulting in a slower and less efficient response to this new foreign antigen. It is under these circumstances that individuals may die directly from the infection. In other situations, individuals may die from untreated secondary infections (in which a second antigen takes advantage of the immune system's already weakened state) or other complications from the illness, such as dehydration.

The activation of the lymphocytes causes other white blood cells of the immune system to become activated and replicate. There are several types of non-antigen specific white blood cells of the immune system including mast cells (basophils) (Figure 3-19), eosinophils (Figure 3-20), polymorphonuclear cells (PMNs) (Figure 3-21), macrophages (monocytes) (Figure 3-22), and natural killer cells. These cells do not look for new foreign antigens specifically; however, they

**Figure 3-19.** The large cells are known as mast cells (also known as basophils). (Photograph courtesy of Burkitt HG, Young B, Daniels VG. *Wheater's Functional Histology: A Text and Color Atlas.* Edinburgh, Scotland: Churchill Livingstone; 1993.)

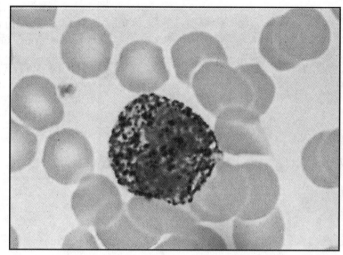

**Figure 3-20.** The large cells are known as eosinophils. (Photograph courtesy of Burkitt HG, Young B, Daniels VG. *Wheater's Functional Histology: A Text and Color Atlas.* Edinburgh, Scotland: Churchill Livingstone; 1993.)

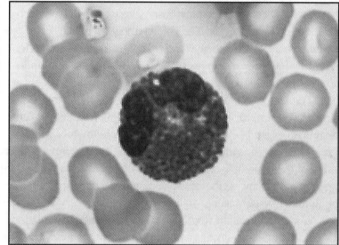

**Figure 3-21.** The large cells are known as polymorphonuclear cells (PMNs) (also referred to as neutrophils). (Photograph courtesy of Burkitt HG, Young B, Daniels VG. *Wheater's Functional Histology: A Text and Color Atlas.* Edinburgh, Scotland: Churchill Livingstone; 1993.)

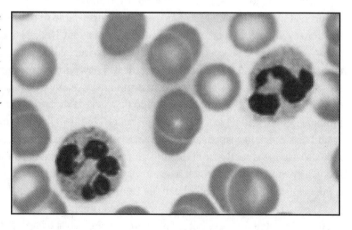

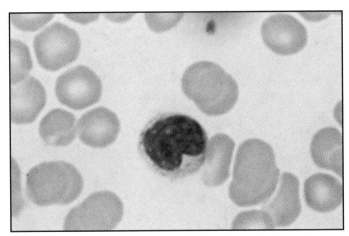

**Figure 3-22.** The large cells are known as macrophages (also referred to as monocytes). (Photograph courtesy of Burkitt HG, Young B, Daniels VG. *Wheater's Functional Histology: A Text and Color Atlas.* Edinburgh, Scotland: Churchill Livingstone; 1993.)

respond to cells that have been "tagged" by antibodies (created by the B-cells for that specific foreign antigen). Once an immune response has been raised and antibody has been formed, many of the infected cells or bacteria will be tagged with the antibody, resulting in destruction by one of the non-specific white blood cells.

Each non-specific white blood cell has a "preference" for the type of antigen it will destroy. Eosinophils are frequently associated with allergic processes (such as pollens), PMNs are found with bacterial infections, and monocytes are associated with viral infections. Lymphocytes may also be detected when there is an infection. Another type of cell, referred to as an inflammatory giant cell (thought to be produced by the fusion of monocytes), is associated with the herpes simplex virus as well as other ocular conditions. Finally, inclusion bodies (the cells which form in response to chlamydial reproduction) will be seen in trachoma infections. Therefore, the presence of a particular white blood cell on a smear gives an indication of the type of infection that is occurring, even if no antigens appear on the slide. This is particularly true in the cases of viruses and allergic conjunctival reactions. These cell bodies can be seen on both Giemsa and Wright stains.

# Reference

1. Centers for Disease Control Morbidity and Mortality Weekly Report. *Epidemic keratoconjunctivitis in an ophthalmology clinic—California.* Atlanta, Ga: Centers for Disease Control; 1990;39:598-601.

# Part II

# Biometry and Echography

# Chapter 4

# Axial Eye Length A-Scans and Intraocular Lens Calculations

## KEY POINTS

- The A-scan axial eye length is a test used to measure the length of the eye.

- The eye length measurement is used in a mathematical formula to derive the power of the intraocular lens (IOL) that will be placed in the patient's eye after cataract extraction.

- There are three A-scan methods used to measure the axial eye length—the immersion method, the slit lamp applanation method, and the hand-held applanation method.

# Axial Eye Length

The axial eye length A-scan, also referred to as biometry, is an important diagnostic procedure in which the exact measurement of the length of the eye is determined. This is such an important procedure that it is the most commonly performed ultrasonographic test of the eye. Both ophthalmologists and ophthalmic medical assistants frequently perform A-scans, so a good understanding of this diagnostic procedure is essential for technical staff working in a busy practice.

The A-scan measurement is used for several reasons, the most common reason being to measure the length of the eye so that proper calculations for the power of an intraocular lens (IOL) can be made prior to cataract surgery. Other reasons why axial eye length A-scans might be performed in the clinical setting include the evaluation of postoperative eye length, eye length growth in children, and asymmetric eye length in individuals with ocular abnormalities such as high myopia. This chapter will focus on A-scan biometry for IOL calculations. However, the techniques used to measure the eye for IOL calculations can also be used for these other applications of biometry.

# Techniques of Axial Eye Length A-Scans

There are three techniques used to perform axial eye length A-scans. These are immersion, slit lamp applanation, and hand-held applanation techniques. (Each will be discussed more fully in later sections.) While the performance of these different A-scans is somewhat dissimilar, the scans they produce are relatively the same. Each technique has its advantages and disadvantages, and most individuals have their own preferences as to which technique to use. The best technique is the one that the operator performs with the greatest accuracy, as this is a measurement in which precision is the most critical factor. Inaccurate axial eye length calculations can result in an IOL with the incorrect power being placed in the eye. This is a very serious complication of cataract surgery and may result in the patient having to undergo further surgery. Therefore, accuracy in performing an A-scan is extremely critical.

# Brief Review

The transducer from the A-scan emits a parallel, point-like sound beam. This results in a one-dimensional representation of the eye that is used for both standard A-scan echography and axial eye length measurements. (See Chapter 5 for the definitions of transducer and ultrasonography.)

The sound beam that is displayed on the monitor looks like a line with a lot of spikes. The spikes represent different tissues in the eye. A spike occurs whenever there is a change in velocity of the sound beam from tissue to tissue. For example, one would expect very few spikes in a normal vitreous, but would expect to see a spike when the sound beam passes from the vitreous to the retina. The interface between the two tissue types results in the noted spike.

The sound beam thus produces a spike at every tissue interface, from left to right. The first tissue spike represents the cornea, and the last tissue spike represents the orbital fat. Other spikes from other tissues within the eye will reside between the anterior (left-most) and posterior (right-most) spikes. These interface spikes are used as guides in measuring the length of the eye.

The height of the spike is based not only on the presence of the interface, but also on how perpendicular the probe is to the tissues being examined. For instance, if the probe for the axial eye length is pointing above the macula, then the height of the retina spike and other tissues noted in the A-scan would be significantly less (ie, shorter) than if the probe were perpendicular to the retina and pointing directly at the macula. Thus the placement of the probe in relationship to the eye in axial eye length measurements is very important.

## Probe Placement

If the eye were round, the A-scan probe could be put on any part of the eye, pointed directly to the other side, and an accurate length of the eye could be calculated. Unfortunately, the eye is egg-shaped, and the longest part of the eye is from the most anterior part of the cornea (generally in the middle of the cornea, over the pupil), to the most posterior part of the eye (generally in the posterior pole at the site of the macula). The full length of the eye includes the sclera, but for the purposes of calculating the length of the eye for an IOL, the most posterior point of interest is the macula. This is because the power of the IOL is calculated so that the light is properly focused on the macula. It is thus necessary to properly align the probe along the visual axis.

Regardless of which of the three techniques is used for axial eye length measurements, probe placement remains the most important aspect of this test. Proper placement results in a relatively accurate calculation of eye length. Improper placement results in the eye being evaluated as shorter than it actually is in the majority of cases. (However, in the event that the probe is directed at the optic nerve, the axial eye length will actually be slightly longer. The scan will look different in that the "retinal" spike, which is actually the nerve head, will be followed by low reflective spikes of the optic nerve and not the typical high reflective spikes of the sclera and orbital fat.)

The properly positioned probe would be directly over the middle of the pupil and pointed directly toward the back of the eye. This results in the sound beam being pointed at the macula. Unfortunately, it is not always possible to know if one is pointing the sound beam directly at the macula. That is where the actual axial eye length A-scan echo pattern is helpful.

## Axial Eye Length Echo Patterns

The echo patterns from most properly aligned axial eye length A-scans are quite similar. It is this similarity in echo patterns that assists in estimating the precision of the measurement. If the A-scan does not look the way it is expected to look, then it can be presumed that the examiner (or the patient) was unable to perform the examination accurately. It is at this point that the examiner should try to repeat the A-scan. The axial eye length measurement should be reliable, meaning that if a second measurement were accurately taken, then the spikes and the eye length calculations would be similar. If it is impossible to obtain a second axial eye length measurement that resembles the first, then it is likely that none of the eye length measurements are actually measuring the length of the eye from the most anterior portion of the cornea to the macula. It is more likely that the probe is improperly positioned. Because of the eye's oblong shape, slight misalignments can mean very improper calculations.

In contact axial eye length A-scans (ie, by slit lamp or hand-held applanation), the first large spike on the far left is that of the anterior cornea. (Remember, A-scans are read from left to right.) This is followed by a spike created by the posterior cornea. (The first spike is actually from the probe/anterior cornea interface.) The anterior and posterior cornea spikes are not separated and actually look like a very "fat" spike (Figure 4-1). The next spike is that of the anterior crystalline lens, followed by a spike from the posterior face of the lens. There is a large section where there is no deviation from the baseline, representing the vitreous cavity. The next interface is at the retina, and this results in a very large spike. A mid-range scleral spike follows this, followed by orbital fat spikes of mid-range height. This is the pattern noted in a phakic eye (see Figure 4-1).

In the immersion method on a phakic eye, the first spike is from the probe/methylcellulose interface. The second spike, from the anterior corneal face, is separated from the posterior corneal spike producing a thin "V" pattern (Figure 4-2). Sometimes the first spike from the probe/methyl-cellulose interface is automatically removed from the display.

In the aphakic eye there are fewer spikes, as the eye does not contain a lens. There is not an anterior lens spike, and there is generally no posterior lens spike. There may be either a posterior capsule or anterior vitreous spike, but the height of this spike is generally not as great as in the phakic eye, as the tissue interface may not be significant (Figure 4-3).

In the pseudophakic eye (an eye with an IOL implanted within it), there will be large artifact spikes following the original IOL spike (Figures 4-4 and 4-5). The A-scans of a person with pseudophakia can be difficult for anyone to evaluate, because it requires turning down the gain (a control on the instrument, to be explained later).

The easiest way to determine if the probe is accurately aligned is to look at the echo patterns. If the corneal, lens, retinal, and scleral spikes are not highly reflective and thus elevated, the alignment is likely wrong. Figure 4-6 shows an axial eye length where the anterior lens, retinal, scleral, and orbital fat echoes are too low. Figure 4-7 shows a scan where the retinal echo is not steeply spiked. Neither scan should be used for calculating axial eye length, since the echoes suggest that the probe is not pointed directly at the macula along the visual axis.

Sometimes it is impossible to obtain the perfect axial eye length measurement due to poor patient cooperation. (A poor scan should never be based on an examiner's limited abilities.) When a patient is uncooperative, the best overall scan should be used. While it is unlikely that the perfect scan will be obtainable under these circumstances, one must do the very best possible to obtain a good scan. When looking at the printouts, use the one with the best retinal spike, and definite scleral and orbital fat spikes. The presence of the retina, sclera, and orbital fat spike complex signifies that the most anterior of those spikes is the retina. Since the retina is the structure where the light will focus after surgery, the relationship between anterior cornea and retina is very important. If the more anterior spikes from the lens and cornea are not as high as you would like, your calculations may not be accurate. However, if the patient is uncooperative and you are trying to determine the general length of the eye from cornea to retina, a high retinal spike with good scleral and fat spikes following is most important.

In all other situations where the patient is cooperative, the spikes must be exactly as expected in order for an accurate axial eye length to be calculated. "Good enough" should be used only on those patients with whom you cannot communicate, and for whom better cooperation is impossible.

## Calculating Axial Eye Lengths with the A-Scan Echo Patterns

An accurate axial eye length can be calculated once a good A-scan has been obtained, and the echo pattern has been measured properly. The accuracy of the axial eye length measurement is based on the assumption that the ultrasonography unit is properly calibrated.

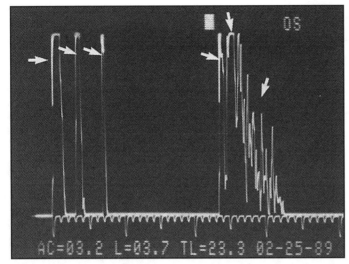

**Figure 4-1.** A classic contact phakic scan, all echoes are clearly defined, tall, and steeply rising. The "fat" spike furthest to thte left is from the cornea. The next spike is from the anterior lens, followed by a large spike from the posterior lens. The flat line represents the clear vitreous. The next set of spikes represent the retina, sclera, and orbital fat. (The scan is read from left to right.) (Reprinted with permission from Kendall CJ. *Ophthalmic Echography.* Thorofare, NJ: SLACK Incorporated; 1990.)

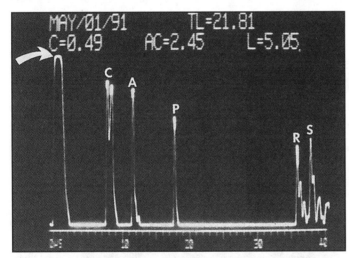

**Figure 4-2.** A classic immersion phakic scan with gates appropriately placed. The gain is reduced and the gates are positioned on the spikes. Note the slight "V" on the corneal spike, representing the anterior and posterior corneal surfaces. Corneal thickness = 0.49 mm; anterior chamber depth = 2.45 mm; lens thickness = 5.05 mm; axial eye length = 21.81 mm. (Reprinted with permission from Byrne SF, Green RL. *Ultrasound of the Eye and Orbit.* St. Louis, Mo: Mosby-Year Book; 1992.)

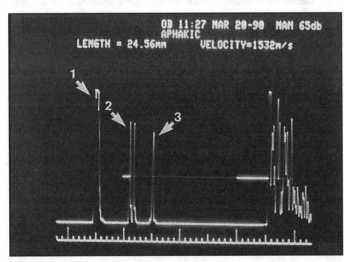

**Figure 4-3.** A classic immersion aphakic scan. Echoes displayed are from probe tip (1), double echo of anterior and posterior cornea (2), and posterior capsule left in the eye after the cataract was removed (3). (Reprinted with permission from Kendall CJ. *Ophthalmic Echography.* Thorofare, NJ: SLACK Incorporated; 1990.)

**Figure 4-4.** A classic pseudophakic axial length scan. The large arrow indicates the IOL echo; smaller three arrows show reverberations. (Reprinted with permission from Kendall CJ. *Ophthalmic Echography.* Thorofare, NJ: SLACK Incorporated; 1990.)

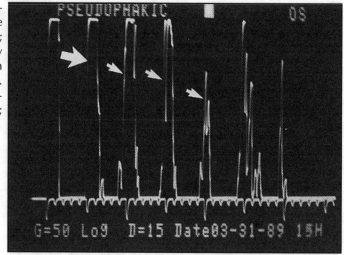

**Figure 4-5.** Another pseudophakic scan with arrows indicating reverbs from IOL. (Reprinted with permission from Kendall CJ. *Ophthalmic Echography.* Thorofare, NJ: SLACK Incorporated; 1990.)

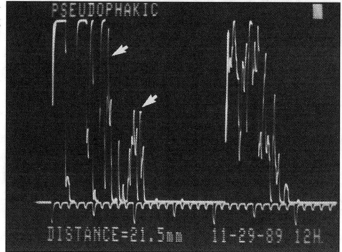

**Figure 4-6.** A poor phakic scan shows insufficient anterior lens, retinal, scleral, and orbital fat echoes. (Reprinted with permission from Kendall CJ. *Ophthalmic Echography.* SLACK Incorporated, 1990.)

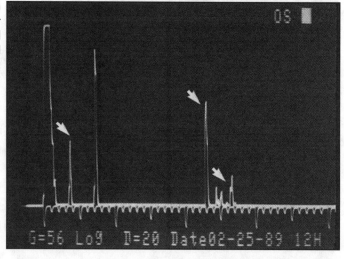

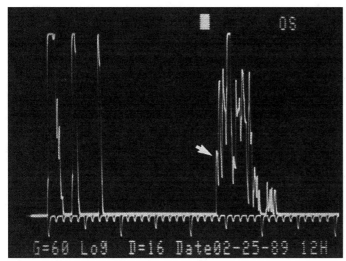

**Figure 4-7.** A poor phakic scan has ragged edge of retinal echo, not steeply rising. (Reprinted with permission from Kendall CJ. *Ophthalmic Echography.* Thorofare, NJ: SLACK Incorporated; 1990.)

## Measuring Gates

Once a reliable, reproducible A-scan has been obtained, the echo pattern is marked with measuring gates or calipers. The measuring gates are marks generated by the computer that are found on the tissue spikes of an A-scan. These marks are used by the computer to make numeric calculations of the length of the eye. The A-scan can be set to either an automatic mode, where the unit automatically places the gates on the spikes that appear appropriate, or to a manual mode, where the examiner has control of gate placement. In manual mode, the gates are moveable, allowing the examiner to move each gate to the appropriate spike. The status of the eye being measured determines the number of gates that will appear on the screen. In a phakic eye there will be four gates, one for the anterior cornea spike, one for the anterior lens spike, one for the posterior lens spike, and one for the retinal spike. If the patient is pseudophakic, three gates will be present—one for the cornea, one for the posterior capsule, and the third for the retina. If the patient is aphakic, there will be only two gates present, one for the anterior cornea and one for the retina.

## What the Patient Needs to Know

- This test will measure the length of your eye. The number will be used in the calculation to determine the strength of the IOL that will be used in your eye.

- The eye will be anesthetized for the test, so you should not feel any discomfort.

- (For the immersion method) A little cup filled with thick tears will be resting on your eye, but it shouldn't be uncomfortable.

- (For the contact method) A little probe will be touching the eye, similar to when we check you for glaucoma. You should not have any discomfort.

- You will be asked to look at a light (or other object) to help you hold your eye straight and still. Try not to move your eye. You may blink now and then, but do not squeeze your eyes.

- Your vision may be somewhat blurry after the test, but that is a normal side effect of the test. (For the immersion method) Your vision will be significantly reduced for about 1 hour.

- Please do not rub your eye for about 1 hour after the examination, because your eye may still be numb.

There are several ways that the gates may appear on the scan, depending on the type of ultrasound unit that is being used. Some of the gates are horizontal bars that are positioned under the echoes being measured, while others are horizontal bars that touch the most left-hand edge of the echo spike. Some gates present a vertical line to the left of the echo, whereas other gates are denoted as small dots that move along the echo spikes. Regardless of how the gates appear, proper placement is essential for accurate axial eye length calculations. In general, the gates are placed at the most left-hand edge of the echo. In the phakic eye, the anterior cornea, the left-hand edge of both the anterior and posterior lens spikes, and the leading edge of the retina are all measured. Figure 4-8 shows measuring gates on a good A-scan. Note that the axial eye length is displayed as 25.70 mm. Figure 4-9 shows the measuring gates in different positions on the same A-scan. Note that the measuring gates on the retina are at a higher point and on the right-hand side of the retinal spike. This incorrect placement of the retinal gate results in an axial eye length calculation of 25.90 mm, which is 0.20 mm longer than the A-scan with the correctly placed gates.

### Tissue Velocity

The echo pattern displayed on the ultrasound monitor provides a graphic representation of the length and structure of the eye. As previously discussed, it is important that a reliable A-scan be recorded and that the spikes be measured properly. There are internal calculations that take place as well. The velocity of the sound wave changes as the beam goes through different tissues within the eye. The aqueous and vitreous humor have tissue velocities of 1,532 meters per second (m/s), soft tissue has velocities of 1,550 m/s, the cornea has a velocity of 1,620 m/s, and the crystalline lens has a velocity of 1,641 m/s. Thus it might be necessary to calculate the overall velocity based on each tissue and its apparent length. To make measuring easier, researchers have calculated an average velocity to be used for axial eye length measurements based on both specific tissue velocity and volume (thickness of the specific tissue being measured). This average velocity (1,548 m/s or sometimes 1,550 m/s) is included in the internal calculations produced by newer ultrasound units used for axial eye length measurements.

Not all eyes are phakic, however; thus it is important to take all of the internal structures into account when velocity calculations are being made. There are controls on the unit that allow the examiner to tell the unit that a phakic, aphakic, or pseudophakic eye is being scanned. By dialing in the eye's status, different velocity calculations will be used in the computation. If a phakic eye is measured using aphakic measurements, then inappropriate calculations and eye measurements will be made.

# Conducting an Axial Eye Length Examination

### Introduction

There are several things common to all axial eye length examinations. The patient needs to be cooperative and fixate on a specific fixation device. (With the immersion technique, the fixation device is often a mark on the ceiling, as the patient will likely be reclined. The applanation-style probe often has a fixation light in it, giving the patient something to look at.) The test does not hurt, as the eye will be anesthetized. Frequently, the fellow eye is tested to verify eye length, as it is unlikely that the two eyes will be significantly different in length. The patient should be tested in a quiet environment, so the best possible A-scan can be obtained.

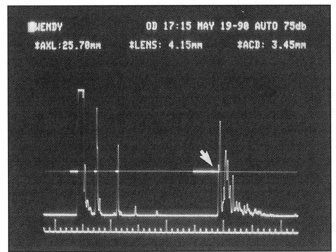

**Figure 4-8.** Correct retinal gate placement is on first part of echo's leading or rising edge. Note measurement of 25.70 mm. (Reprinted with permission from Kendall CJ. *Ophthalmic Echography*. Thorofare, NJ: SLACK Incorporated; 1990.)

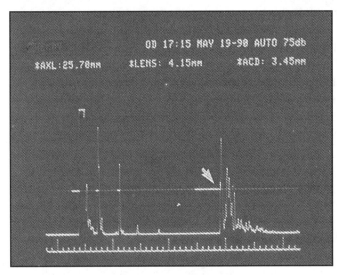

**Figure 4-9.** Incorrect retinal gate placement on the higher part of the echo past steeply rising edge shows an increase in measurement of 0.20 mm. (Reprinted with permission from Kendall CJ. *Ophthalmic Echography*. Thorofare, NJ: SLACK Incorporated; 1990.)

The A-scan is displayed on a monitor on the ultrasound unit. The unit can be set to automatically determine which scan is "correct" and freeze the frame, or the examiner can decide which scan is accurate. As the probe moves on the eye, the A-scan echoes move about. If the ultrasound unit is on the automatic freezing mode, the unit will freeze the image when the echo spikes fall within a certain range. In the manual mode a foot pedal is pressed when a scan looks correct to the examiner, freezing the image on the monitor. The gates can then be moved into the correct place, and axial eye length measurements are produced on the screen. The image is either photographed or printed out.

The most proficient examiners will usually choose the manual mode, while the beginners will choose the automatic freeze mode. It is important for any examiner to understand what the A-scan echo patterns should look like and not rely solely on the computer for making the decision as to whether or not an A-scan echo pattern is valid.

Once the examination is over, the instruments will need to be cleaned. The scleral shells used in the immersion method (described next) can first be rinsed off with tap water to remove the excess methylcellulose, then cleaned with alcohol swabs. The shell should be vigorously swabbed for several minutes. (An alternative method is to soak the scleral shell in a 3% hydrogen peroxide solution for 5 minutes, followed by a 5 minute soak in sterile saline. The shell should then be towel dried.) Once swabbed, the shell should be rinsed again with sterile saline or distilled water.

A solid-tipped A-scan probe can be wiped with an alcohol pad and rinsed with sterile saline or distilled water. If the A-scan probe has a membrane tip, certain cleaning solutions may need to be avoided, as they may be absorbed by the pores of some membranes and damage other membranes. Individuals should check the manual or contact the manufacturer to find out the recommended disinfection procedure for a particular probe. (See Appendix B for more information on Universal Precautions.)

## Immersion Technique

As its name implies, the immersion technique is one in which the probe does not directly touch the cornea. Instead, the probe is immersed in an artificial tear solution. This method provides the examiner with the exact position of the anterior corneal spike in reference to the probe.

In the immersion method, a scleral shell is placed on the anesthetized cornea, supported by the lids. There are several varieties of scleral shells available on the market (Figures 4-10 to 4-12). The shell is fit onto the eye, filled with a solution (most frequently 2.5% methylcellulose), and then the probe is placed into the liquid without touching the cornea.

After anesthetic has been instilled in the eye, the patient is placed in a reclined position. He or she is asked to look straight ahead as the shell is placed on the cornea. The upper-most edge of the shell fits under the upper lid, and the lower-most edge of the shell slides under the lower lid. The shell is filled with methylcellulose. Care should be taken to avoid air bubbles, as these can disrupt echographic patterns. The patient is asked not to move excessively, as excessive movement reduces the reliability of the examination. Performing the measurement in a quiet examination room assists in this process.

The patient is given a fixation light to watch with both eyes open. This gives the examiner some idea of where the covered cornea is looking. The probe is placed in the shell to be parallel with it, and perpendicular to the eyeball.

The fact that the probe is not directly on the cornea gives the examiner several advantages. For starters, the first peak in the scan is from the probe/methylcellulose interface. This is followed by a section that is absent of spikes. This represents the area of the shell that is filled with methylcellulose but neither touched by the probe or the cornea. The second major spike comes from the anterior section of the cornea. (In some ultrasound units, the probe/methylcellulose interface is not shown, thus the first spike will be the anterior cornea. Check the manual to determine if the probe/methylcellulose spike is or is not present on your scans.)

The advantage of the immersion method over the contact variety is that there is no false distance from the probe and the cornea, which sometimes exists with the contact method when the probe does not rest properly on the cornea. (In the contact method, if the probe rests on a layer of methylcellulose and not directly on the cornea, the length of the eye will be artificially long.) There is also no artificial shortening of the globe that sometimes occurs with the contact method when the probe is pushed too hard on the cornea. The corneal spike in an immersion axial eye length is about the most accurate that can be produced, given that the patient is otherwise cooperative.

Once several reproducible scans have been acquired, the test can be considered complete. (It is best to obtain more than one scan, just in case the quality of one is not to your standards. It

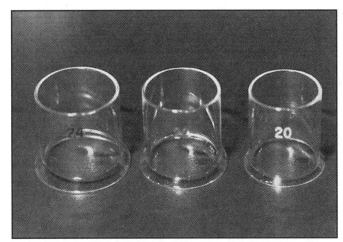

**Figure 4-10.** Immersion shells, set of three different sizes. (Reprinted with permission from Kendall CJ. *Ophthalmic Echography*. Thorofare, NJ: SLACK Incorporated; 1990.)

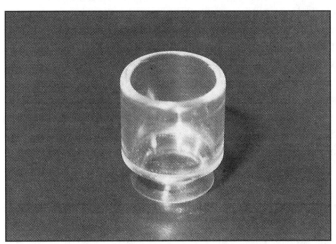

**Figure 4-11.** Immersion shell, one size fits all. (Reprinted with permission from Kendall CJ. *Ophthalmic Echography*. Thorofare, NJ: SLACK Incorporated; 1990.)

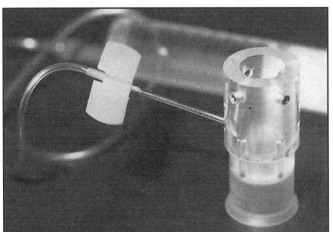

**Figure 4-12.** Immersion shell, custom made for a specific probe with side port to inject fluid. (Reprinted with permission from Kendall CJ. *Ophthalmic Echography*. Thorofare, NJ: SLACK Incorporated; 1990.)

would be very unfortunate to have to repeat the entire process on a patient whom you have just cleaned up.) After the scan has been completed, the shell is removed (have the patient look up when you do this). Have a tissue on hand to collect the excessive methylcellulose solution from the shell or the solution will run down the patient's cheek. The patient's eye should be rinsed with a sterile unpreserved saline solution (not from an aerosol can), and the patient should be given some type of artificial tears for later use, just in case the eye feels uncomfortable.

## Slit Lamp Applanation

A-scan biometry is most often performed using the slit lamp applanation technique. This method is considered easier to perform by many, and patients are more familiar with this technique because it resembles the apparatus used for applanation tonometry. (Despite the fact that the examiner and the patient may feel this is an easier technique for axial eye length evaluations, there are several drawbacks to using this method. These will be addressed in a later section.)

Either one of two methods can be used for the applanation technique. In the first method, the A-scan probe is placed on the slit lamp in the holder for the Goldmann applanation tonometer tip. If the slit lamp is not fitted with a Goldmann tonometer apparatus, an A-scan adapter can be placed on the slit lamp instead. The tonometer knob must be adjusted away from the zero mark until the probe is no longer shifted back. This allows the probe to gently but constantly touch the cornea at an angle that is parallel to the front of the eye and perpendicular to the back of the eye.

After a local anesthetic is instilled, the patient is instructed to put his or her chin in the chin rest. The forehead should rest firmly against the forehead bar, and the bar should be positioned in the middle of the patient's forehead. The chin should fit all the way forward, but should not fit too far forward or too far back on the chin rest (Figures 4-13 and 4-14). The probe is moved forward toward the patient's eye using the joystick. The patient is instructed not to move his or her head, and to keep the eyes wide open. The probe should gently rest on the cornea without indenting it (which will make the axial eye length too short), and without leaving a space between the probe tip and the cornea (which will make the axial eye length too long) (Figures 4-15 through 4-19). The examiner should view the patient's eye quickly to verify the correct position, and should then view the monitor until appropriate echo spikes are visible. The positioning of the probe is done by the joystick in a manner similar to moving a tonometer tip. Small movements should be used when refining the position of the probe on the cornea. When looking at the echo pattern on the applanation A-scan, remember that the cornea spike will be "fat" and will not display the separate spikes for the anterior and posterior corneal surfaces as do the immersion echo patterns.

One big disadvantage to using this device is that the probe is handled excessively as it is placed into and removed from the slit lamp for each measurement. A possible solution is to use one examination room and slit lamp only for A-scan biometry. However, in a busy clinic this may or may not be an effective use of time and space. To address this problem, a freestanding chin rest (ie, without a slit lamp) has been designed on which the A-scan probe can be mounted. The chin rest is similar to that of the slit lamp and the applanation A-scan probe is moved by a joystick. This chin rest apparatus is commercially available for virtually all A-scan biometry units.

## Hand-Held Applanation

The third and final means by which to obtain axial eye lengths is by the hand-held applanation method. This method uses a probe that is similar to the one used for the slit lamp applana-

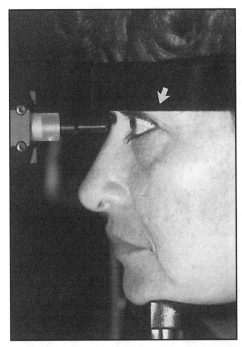

**Figure 4-13.** Incorrect position—forehead band low. (Reprinted with permission from Kendall CJ. *Ophthalmic Echography*. Thorofare, NJ: SLACK Incorporated; 1990.)

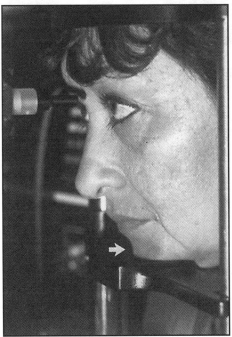

**Figure 4-14.** Incorrect position—chin back. (Reprinted with permission from Kendall CJ. *Ophthalmic Echography*. Thorofare, NJ: SLACK Incorporated; 1990.)

**Figure 4-15.** Patient has just blinked and probe is slowly moved toward cornea. (Reprinted with permission from Kendall CJ. *Ophthalmic Echography.* Thorofare, NJ: SLACK Incorporated; 1990.)

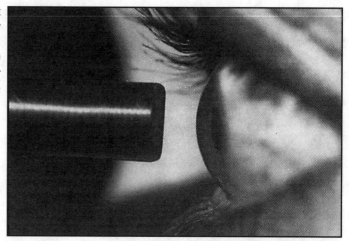

**Figure 4-16.** Solid A-scan probe is gently in contact with the film of the cornea. (Reprinted with permission from Kendall CJ. *Ophthalmic Echography.* Thorofare, NJ: SLACK Incorporated; 1990.)

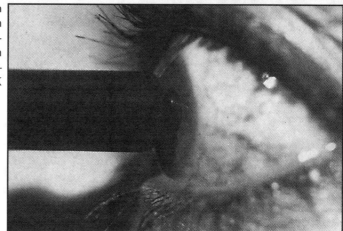

**Figure 4-17.** Correct applanation pressure to cornea–probe tip is in gentle contact with the cornea. (Reprinted with permission from Kendall CJ. *Ophthalmic Echography.* Thorofare, NJ: SLACK Incorporated; 1990.)

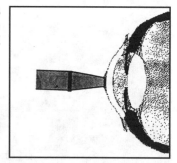

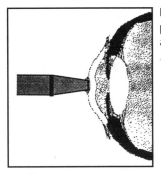

**Figure 4-18.** Too much applanation pressure compresses the cornea, producing falsely shallow anterior chamber depth and falsely short axial length. (Reprinted with permission from Kendall CJ. *Ophthalmic Echography*. Thorofare, NJ: SLACK Incorporated; 1990.)

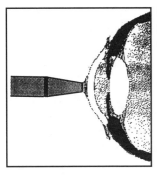

**Figure 4-19.** Too little applanation pressure–fluid bridge between probe tip and cornea causes falsely deep anterior chamber depth and falsely long axial length. (Reprinted with permission from Kendall CJ. *Ophthalmic Echography*. Thorofare, NJ: SLACK Incorporated; 1990.)

tor. Instead of the probe resting in a fixed mount, however, the probe is held in the examiner's hand. The probe is placed on the anesthetized eye, and the patient is instructed to look in the direction of a fixation light. The probe must still be kept perpendicular to the back of the eye, while at the same time aligning with the visual axis to the macula. The examiner must make sure that the probe rests gently on the cornea without indenting it.

This technique may be quite useful in situations where the patient is bed-bound, or in individuals who are overly frightened about having a big scleral shell put on their eye. Generally speaking, however, this is the least efficient method and the one that has the greatest potential for producing erroneous measurements. Small movements to realign the probe may be difficult for even the most proficient of examiners.

## IOL Power Calculations

The main reason for obtaining axial eye length measurements is to determine the power of the IOL that will be placed in the patient's eye during cataract surgery. The postoperative anterior chamber depth (in millimeters), from the anterior-most aspect of the cornea to the anterior surface of the pseudophakic lens, must be estimated. This estimation is based on the length of the preoperative eye. However, the axial eye length measurement is only one of several numeric values that must be obtained in order for the appropriate IOL to be selected. The radius of the cornea in millimeters or the corneal power in diopters also needs to be acquired (via keratometry, called K readings). Once these values have been established, and the postoperative refractive error has been agreed upon (some patients prefer to have a plano refractive error, while others desire a slight myopic refractive error), the IOL power calculations can be made.

There are several formulas that have been scientifically tested by ophthalmologists working in this field. (The formulas are generally named after the ophthalmologist who invented the particular formula.) The formulas differ only slightly from one another mathematically speaking, and most offer similar and reliable results. The formulas are available on computer programs, calculators, or the ultrasound unit itself. Each ophthalmologist has his or her preferred formula for calculating IOL powers. These preferences may be based on the type of IOL that is being used, or on prior experience with the formula. The formula that is preferred by the ophthalmologist may be the one that his or her mentor preferred.

Most A-scan biometry units have built-in mini-processors so that IOL power calculations can be processed by the biometer and printed out for permanent record. The computer can perform several types of computations including IOL powers to obtain emmetropia and IOL powers to obtain specific refractive errors. The calculations can be performed using different IOL formulas, thus giving the ophthalmologist numerous choices when selecting IOL powers.

IOL power calculations are obviously very important. Several factors in the A-scan itself may result in inappropriate IOL powers. Technicians should be concerned if the axial eye length is under 22 mm or over 25 mm. Differences of more than 0.3 mm between the eyes are also suspect. If any of these situations occur with axial eye length measurements, then the A-scan should be repeated (perhaps by a different operator). Inaccurate K readings can also result in improper IOL power calculations. The technician should be concerned (and probably repeat the reading) if the K readings are less than 40 D or greater than 47 D. Also, the K reading should be compared to the refractometric measurement. While some discrepancy may exist due to lenticular astigmatism, the K readings and refraction should more or less agree in axis and cylinder amount. If any of the above situations occur, it is essential to make the ophthalmologist aware of the problem.

# Suggested Reading

Shammas, HJ. *Intraocular Lens Power Calculations: Avoiding the Errors*. Glendale, Calif: The News Circle Publishing House, 1996.

Chapter 5

# Diagnostic A- and B-Scan Ultrasonography

**KEY POINTS**

- The use of ocular ultrasound allows for the examination of the structures of the eye, even when there is dense opacification of the media.

- The A-scan produces a one-dimensional view of the eye.

- The B-scan produces a two-dimensional view of the eye.

- Abnormalities, such as retinal or choroidal detachments, intraocular tumors, metallic foreign bodies, and extraocular muscle thickening can be detected by means of ultrasound.

Over the past several decades the usefulness of diagnostic ultrasonography has become more and more apparent. Ocular ultrasonography is indicated for the evaluation of the eye with opacities where the view of either the anterior or posterior segments is limited, as well as in eyes with clear media where structures are apparently abnormal (as in the case of tumors). This section will introduce the reader to the general principals of diagnostic A- and B-scan ultrasonography, describe the basic techniques of performing A- and B-scan ultrasonographic examinations, and give indications and examples of A- and B-scan ultrasonography. This is intended to be introductory material. Individuals who are interested in a more extensive treatment of the subject are referred to the book *Ultrasound of the Eye and Orbit* by Sandra Frazier Burne and Ronald L. Green, MD, published by Mosby, St. Louis, 1992.

# Basic Principles

The ultrasonographic technique that is used today in ophthalmology is referred to as Standardized Echography. (Echography and ultrasonography are generally used interchangeably, but the term Standardized Echography denotes a particular examination technique.) Standardized Echography is based on work by Karl Ossoinig.[1] Ossoinig believed that standardized techniques and instrumentation were essential if all examiners were going to be able to provide comparable and reproducible results. Without comparable results, each patient would have to be followed by the same physician, in the same laboratory, using the same instrument for all examinations. This would greatly reduce the usefulness of ocular ultrasonography. Ossoinig believed that echographers could use others' findings, if all of the scans were done similarly. Ossoinig developed the first standardized A-scan instrument and later developed a standardized contact B-scan instrument. He also developed standardized examination techniques to be used with both instruments. These techniques eventually developed into what is known as Standardized Echography, which was quickly accepted by the ophthalmic community. The Standardized Echography examination techniques and clinical findings, which includes the use of both standardized A- and B-scan echography, will be described later in this chapter.

Ultrasound is an inaudible acoustic (sound) wave that consists of oscillating particles. Ultrasound waves have a frequency of greater than 20,000 oscillations per second (20 KHz). For Standardized Echography, the frequencies generally range from 8 to 10 million cycles per second (8 to 10 MHz). These very high frequencies produce very short wavelengths, in the range of 0.2 mm. This allows for excellent resolution of the small structures of the eye and orbit.

All clinical echography depends on instrumentation that both emits an ultrasonographic wave then detects and processes the returning waves (Figure 5-1). All echographic instruments contain piezo-electrical materials such as quartz crystals or ceramic plates called transducers. (Ultrasound transducers that are built into hand-held units are called probes. The transducer is housed at the very tip where the probe touches the eye.) The transducer emits ultrasonographic waves, also referred to as sound beams. As the ultrasound wave passes through the tissues of the eye, part of the wave is reflected back to the transducer. This reflected wave is referred to as an echo. The echoes are produced when two adjacent tissues have different sound velocities (speed at which sound travels). For example, when the ultrasound wave goes through a normal vitreous, there is no change in sound velocity and there is no echo reflected back to the transducer. However, when the ultrasound wave reaches the retina, there is a change in sound velocity, thus resulting in an echo that is reflected back to the transducer. The greater the difference in velocity between the adjacent tissues, the greater the reflected echo. The reflected echoes are detected by the transducer, then amplified, and displayed on the screen of the ultrasound unit.

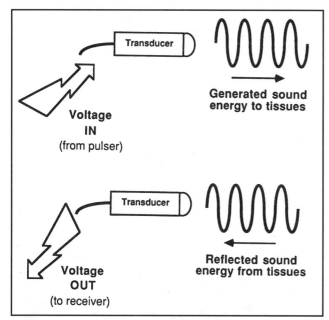

**Figure 5-1.** Ultrasound transducers are ceramic plates that transform electricity into sound waves and sound waves into electricity. (Reprinted with permission from Kendall CJ. *Ophthalmic Echography.* Thorofare, NJ: SLACK Incorporated; 1990.)

In A-scan ultrasonography, the transducer emits a parallel, point-like sound beam (Figure 5-2). This results in a one-dimensional representation of the eye. The display looks like a line that has a lot of spikes on it. The spikes represent echoes from different tissues within the eye. In the normal eye using the contact method, the first spike represents the corneal artifact, followed by the second spike that indicates the anterior face of the lens. The next spike comes from the posterior face of the lens. In the normal eye, there is then a length of space where the line does not spike. This represent the vitreous. The final spike is from the back of the eye and the adjacent fat of the orbit (Figure 5-3). The structures of the eye in A-scan ultrasonography are always read from left to right.

In B-scan ultrasonography, the transducer oscillates back and forth, resulting in a two-dimensional picture that looks like black and white photograph (Figure 5-4). The echoes are depicted as white structural images that resemble portions of the eye, such as the ones depicted in Figure 5-5. The picture represents a "slice" through the portion of the eye being examined. The "slice" may represent either a horizontal or vertical view of the eye. In B-scan ultrasonography, the results allow for a topographic evaluation of the structures of the eye and orbit.

## Standardized Echography Examination Techniques

Standardized Echography consists of specific examination techniques that allow for the thorough evaluation of the eye. The type of examination that is conducted is based on the reason for the examination. The contact method, where the probe is placed directly on the cornea, is used when the posterior segment is examined. The first real echo that is seen using this technique comes from the iris, as the reflection from the cornea (or lid, if the eye is closed) results in a large echographic artifact. The immersion technique is used when the anterior segment needs to be evaluated. In the immersion technique, a clear plastic tube about the size of the cornea and about 1 centimeter high is placed over the anesthetized eye (Figure 5-6). The tube is filled with

**Figure 5-2.** The stationary transducer in an A-scan produces a one-dimensional display. (Reprinted with permission from Kendall CJ. *Ophthalmic Echography.* Thorofare, NJ: SLACK Incorporated; 1990.)

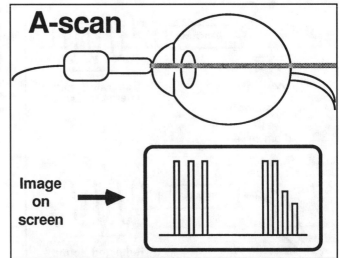

**Figure 5-3.** The characteristic echoes in an axial eye length A-scan are cornea (C), anterior lens (A), posterior lens (P), retina (R), sclera (S), and orbital fat (F). (Reprinted with permission from Kendall CJ. *Ophthalmic Echography.* Thorofare, NJ: SLACK Incorporated; 1990.)

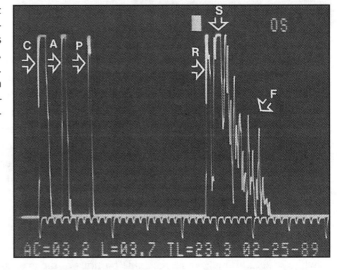

**Figure 5-4.** The moving ceramic transducer inside the B-scan probe sends out an array of individual sound beams. The reflections from each beam is organized and displayed as a two-dimensional image. (Reprinted with permission from Kendall CJ. *Ophthalmic Echography.* Thorofare, NJ: SLACK Incorporated; 1990.)

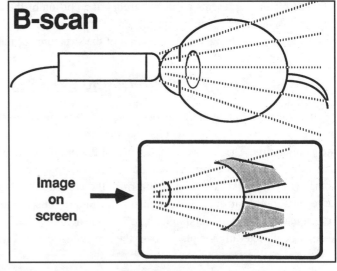

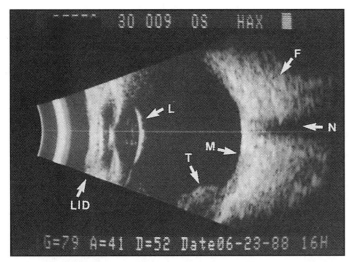

**Figure 5-5.** This B-scan directed through the horizontal axis of the eye shows the eyelid (LID), posterior lens (L), a tumor (T), the macula (M), optic nerve (N), and orbital fat (F). (Reprinted with permission from Kendall CJ. *Ophthalmic Echography.* Thorofare, NJ: SLACK Incorporated; 1990.)

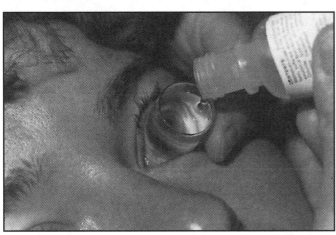

**Figure 5-6.** Fill shell almost to top to allow for changes in probe depth. (Reprinted with permission from Kendall CJ. *Ophthalmic Echography.* Thorofare, NJ: SLACK Incorporated; 1990.)

## What the Patient Needs to Know

- This test is used to evaluate the structures of your eye, as well as the surrounding structures. Pictures will be taken of these structures to make sure that no abnormalities exist.

- The eye will be numbed for the test, so you should not feel any discomfort.

- (For the immersion method—to evaluate the anterior chamber) A little cup filled with thick tears will be resting on your eye, but it shouldn't be uncomfortable.

- (For the contact method—to evaluate the posterior chamber) A probe will be touching the eye (or lid) and it may feel wet, as a small amount of thick tears are placed on the end of the probe. You should not have any discomfort, but may feel a slight vibration and/or slight pressure from the moving probe.

- You will be asked to look in several directions. It is important that you maintain fixation while these different areas of your eye are being evaluated.

- Try not to blink or move the eyes except when asked.

- Your vision may be somewhat blurry after the test, but that is a normal side effect of the test. (For the immersion method) Your vision will be significantly reduced for about one hour.

- Please do not rub your eye for about one hour after the examination, because your eye may still be numb.

**Figure 5-7.** "Mini-immersion" scan uses the same axial length. A B-probe is gently placed on the top rim of a filled shell. The empty space at the beginning of the scan corresponds to the fluid in the shell. Cornea (C), lens (L), ciliary body (CB), and optic nerve (N) are readily seen. This technique provides greater resolution in the anterior segment. (Reprinted with permission from Kendall CJ. *Ophthalmic Echography*. Thorofare, NJ: SLACK Incorporated; 1990.)

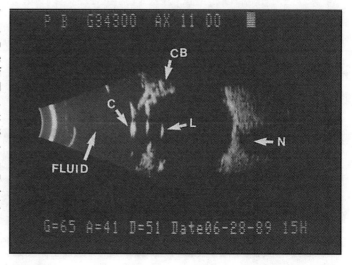

2.5% sterile methylcellulose and the probe is placed into the tube. This results in the first echoes coming from the anterior cornea, as the methylcellulose and cornea have different sound velocities. (Remember, when the probe is placed directly on the cornea, there is a large probe/corneal artifact. This artifact is so large that the cornea cannot be evaluated.) The methylcellulose/anterior surface cornea interface results in a clean echo that can be evaluated. The posterior cornea, iris, and lens also produce echoes that can be easily recognized by this technique. Therefore, the immersion technique allows for full examination of the structures of the anterior chamber (Figure 5-7). Both the immersion and contact techniques can be used with either the A- or B-scan probes.

The evaluation techniques are similar between A- and B-scans; however, because the two types of transducers perform different functions, the results from the two examinations are different. Also, the immersion and the contact method use similar testing parameters. A methodical and systematic evaluation of all quadrants of the eye is necessary in order to perform Standardized Echography.

## Standardized A-Scan Techniques

The A-scan probe sends a single sound wave from the transducer tip to the back of the eye. The position of the probe determines which part of the eye is being examined. The instrument is adjusted so that the probe setting is on "tissue sensitivity." The patient is asked to look up and the probe is placed on the limbus in the 6 o'clock position. The probe is moved from the limbus to the fornix, while the patient continues to look up. This provides information from the more posterior part of the 12 o'clock meridian, to a more anterior part of the 12 o'clock meridian (Figure 5-8). The seven remaining meridians are tested, with the probe on the side opposite the patient's position of gaze. This results in a full screen of the back of the eye. Next, the sensitivity is turned down about 24 decibels below that of "tissue sensitivity." The patient is again tested, using all eight meridians, at this new setting. This allows for an evaluation of more subtle defects that could not be detected when the setting was at the "tissue sensitivity" level. (See also Figures 5-18 through 5-23.)

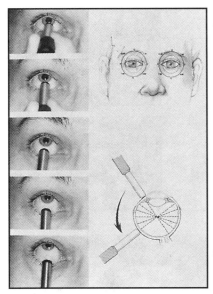

**Figure 5-8.** A-scan screening of the posterior segment. As the patient looks up, probe is shifted from limbus to fornix along the 6 o'clock meridian (thereby examining the 12 o'clock meridian). This limbus to fornix shifting is performed in eight meridians to screen the entire posterior segment. (Reprinted with permission from Green RL, Bryne SF. Diagnostic ophthalmic ultrasound. In: Ryan SJ, ed. *Retina.* St. Louis, Mo: CV Mosby Co; 1989.)

## Standardized B-Scan Techniques

B-scan echography uses the same eight meridians for screening the back of the eye. However, since the B-scan probe provides a two-dimensional image, the position of the probe determines which way the beam is oriented and what part of the eye is being evaluated. So, before the examination techniques for B-scan are explained, a review of probe positioning is necessary.

The probe has a specific orientation that is determined by a mark on the side of the probe. The white mark corresponds to the top of the echographic image that is displayed on the screen. For example, if the patient is looking straight ahead and the probe is placed on the eye with the mark facing the nose, the image on the screen will represent the back of the eye, with the top portion representing the nasal portion of the globe. If the probe is placed on the eye with the mark facing up, the top portion of the echographic image will represent the superior portion of the globe.

### Probe Positions

The three main probe positions used in B-scan ultrasonography are transverse, longitudinal, and axial. Each will be discussed briefly.

#### Transverse Scans

The transverse position is used to scan the four quadrants of the eye. This is done using horizontal, vertical, and oblique probe orientations. The probe is placed on the eye to evaluate it from the posterior pole to a more anterior aspect. For example, when evaluating either the superior or inferior quadrant, the examiner uses a horizontal transverse approach and views everything from the posterior pole to the ora serrata (of either the superior or inferior aspect of the globe). To view the superior aspect, the probe is placed on the limbus in the 6 o'clock position while the patient is looking upward (Figure 5-9). The probe mark is always oriented nasally when a horizontal transverse scan is performed, so the upper part of the scan represents the nasal aspect of the eye.

To view either the nasal or temporal quadrants, a vertical transverse probe placement is used. For example, to view the nasal quadrant of the right eye, the probe is placed on the temporal side at the limbus (9 o'clock position) while the patient is looking nasally. The probe mark is always oriented superiorly when doing a vertical transverse scan, so the upper part of the scan represents the top portion of the eye (Figure 5-10).

**Figure 5-9.** Horizontal transverse scan through superior equatorial portion of globe. *Top*, normal globe; *bottom* elevated lesion. Probe marker is oriented nasally. (Reprinted with permission from Green RL, Bryne SF. Diagnostic ophthalmic ultrasound. In: Ryan SJ, ed. *Retina*. St. Louis, Mo: CV Mosby Co; 1989.)

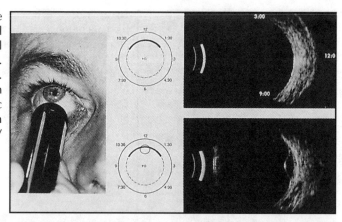

**Figure 5-10.** Vertical transverse scan where probe marker is superior and the probe is placed temporally to image nasally. The patient looks away from the probe. (Reprinted with permission from Kendall CJ. *Ophthalmic Echography*. Thorofare, NJ: SLACK Incorporated; 1990.)

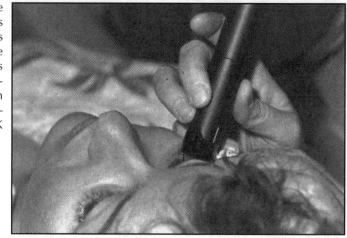

In some cases oblique views may be necessary. In such instances, the patient is asked to look either up and to the right (1:30), down and to the right (4:30), down and to the left (7:30), or up and to the left (10:30). The probe is placed on the limbus opposite to the direction of gaze. The probe mark is always oriented toward the upper portion of the globe, so the top of the scan represents to top portion of the eye. In all of the transverse scans, the sound beam does not go through the lens, as the probe is placed on the eye to avoid it.

**Longitudinal Scans**

The longitudinal position is perpendicular to the transverse approach. The probe is placed on the patient's eye with the mark pointing in the direction that the patient is looking (Figures 5-11 through 5-14). If we examine the superior quadrant using the longitudinal approach, the probe is placed in the 6 o'clock position and pointed to the 12 o'clock position (Figure 5-15). (The probe is always *placed* in the opposite meridian of that being tested, with the *mark* pointing toward the meridian to be tested, as described above.) The transducer moves along the 12 o'clock meridian, ranging from the optic nerve up to the ora serrata. The optic nerve appears on the bottom of the ultrasound screen, and the superior aspect of the eye appears on the top. (When the longitudinal position is used, the optic nerve always appears on the bottom of the screen.) This view gives information about the anterior/posterior aspect of any observed lesion. Again, because of probe position, the sound beam does not go through the lens.

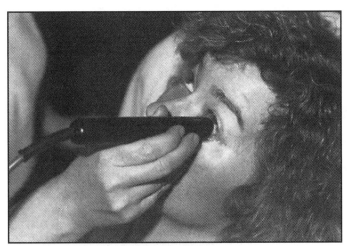

**Figure 5-11.** A longitudinal scan with the probe marker toward the cornea and the patient looking away. Probe is placed at the 6:00 limbus to image the 12:00 radius from optic nerve to ciliary body; image labeled L 12:00. (Reprinted with permission from Kendall CJ. *Ophthalmic Echography.* Thorofare, NJ: SLACK Incorporated; 1990.)

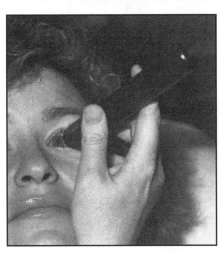

**Figure 5-12.** Another longitudinal scan with the probe marker toward the cornea and the patient looking away. Probe is placed at the 3:00 limbus to image the 9:00 radius from optic nerve to ciliary body; image labeled L 9:00. (Reprinted with permission from Kendall CJ. *Ophthalmic Echography.* Thorofare, NJ: SLACK Incorporated; 1990.)

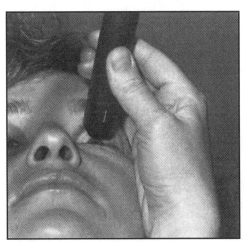

**Figure 5-13.** A longitudinal scan with the probe marker toward the cornea and the patient looking away. Probe is placed at the 12:00 limbus to image the 6:00 radius from optic nerve to ciliary body; image labeled L 6:00. (Reprinted with permission from Kendall CJ. *Ophthalmic Echography.* Thorofare, NJ: SLACK Incorporated; 1990.)

**Figure 5-14.** This is the most important longitudinal scan. The probe is placed at the 9:00 limbus to image the 3:00 radius from optic nerve to ciliary body; image labeled L 3:00. This probe position will image the macula. On the right eye the longitudinal macula scan is L 9:00 with the probe placed at the 3:00 limbus, marker toward cornea. (Reprinted with permission from Kendall CJ. *Ophthalmic Echography.* Thorofare, NJ: SLACK Incorporated; 1990.)

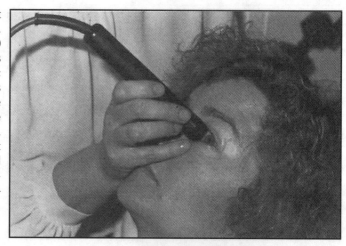

**Figure 5-15.** Longitudinal scan of 12 o'clock meridian. *Top,* normal globe; *bottom,* elevated lesion. Probe marker is oriented toward the cornea *ON,* optic nerve; *P,* posterior; *A,* anterior. (Reprinted with permission from Green RL, Bryne SF. Diagnostic ophthalmic ultrasound. In: Ryan SJ, ed. *Retina.* St. Louis, Mo: CV Mosby Co; 1989.)

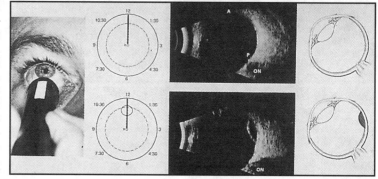

### Axial Scans

The axial position is designed to evaluate the different meridians of the eye in relationship to the lens of the eye. The patient looks straight ahead and the probe is placed directly on the cornea (Figure 5-16). The difference between this technique and the longitudinal is that the sound beam passes through the lens. The position of the probe results in the optic nerve being in the center of the screen. This is the least effective method to evaluate the posterior segment because of the sound attenuation caused by the lens.

## Labeling

During the examination, the A- and B-scan images are either printed out or photographed. The image is recorded when it is representative of the structure of the eye under investigation. The different probe positions allow for the complete examination of the eye, thus resulting in a topographic representation of the eye.

In order for the A- and B-scan images to provide this critical information, they must be labeled properly. Labeling is generally based on both the probe position (transverse, longitudinal, or axial), and the location of the probe on the eye (probe is on the 12 o'clock limbus pointing toward 6 o'clock, in the direction of the posterior pole). The transverse scan is labeled based on the meridian being examined as well as the actual position in which the probe is pointing, such

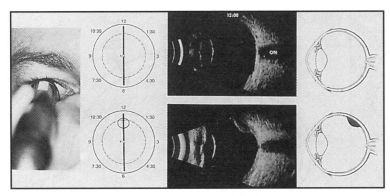

**Figure 5-16.** Vertical axial scan. *Top,* normal globe; *bottom,* elevated lesion. *ON,* optic nerve. (Reprinted with permission from Green RL, Bryne SF. Diagnostic ophthalmic ultrasound. In: Ryan SJ, ed. *Retina.* St. Louis, Mo: CV Mosby Co; 1989.)

as toward the posterior pole, resulting in a label of 12:00 P or toward the equator resulting in a label of 12:00 E (Figure 5-17 through 5-23). The longitudinal scan is labeled "L" for probe position and the meridian that is being examined (such as 4:00) for a label of L 4:00. The horizontal and vertical axial positions are the easiest to label (HAX for horizontal axial and VAX for vertical axial). The oblique axials are labeled 10:30 AX or 1:30 AX, for example. (Remember the probe is pointed upward on axial scans, so the oblique axials will always be somewhere between 9:00 to 3:00.)

# B-Scan Examination

In Standardized Echography (A- or B-scan), each examination should be performed exactly the same way on every patient. This assures that the topographic evaluation is consistent and can be replicated on another date or in another laboratory. The patient is placed in a comfortable, generally supine, position. The eye is anesthetized to reduce potential discomfort.

For a B-scan, the globe is first evaluated using the transverse approach to examine the superior portion of the globe. The patient is instructed to look up in the 12 o'clock position and the B-scan probe is placed directly on the limbus at the 6 o'clock position with the mark pointed toward the patient's nose. The probe remains at the 6 o'clock position but is moved from the limbus to the fornix while the tip of the probe is still pointing toward 12 o'clock. (The patient continues to hold the 12 o'clock gaze.) This results in an examination of the superior portion of the globe from the superior-posterior fundus (when the probe was on the limbus) to a more peripheral area of the superior globe (as the probe is shifted toward the fornix) (Figure 5-24).

The nasal portion of the globe is examined next. The patient is asked to look medially while the probe is placed on the temporal limbus. The probe is oriented vertically with the mark pointed toward 12 o'clock. Again, the probe is moved from the limbus to the temporal fornix while the patient continues to look nasally. This results in an evaluation of the nasal half of the globe. This procedure is repeated in a similar manner for both the inferior and temporal quadrants of the globe. When the inferior quadrant is tested, the probe marker is pointed toward the nose. When the temporal quadrant is tested, the probe marker is pointed up, in the 12 o'clock position.

After the globe has been fully evaluated using the transverse method, the eye is evaluated from both the horizontal and vertical axial positions. The probe is placed directly over the cornea while the patient looks straight ahead. When the vertical axial position is tested, the mark on the probe is facing the 12 o'clock position. When the horizontal axial position is tested, the mark on the probe is facing the nasal position (3 o'clock on the right eye, and 9 o'clock on the left eye).

**Figure 5-17.** Keep a copy of this labeling diagram available during every examination for assistance in determining the area being imaged. (Reprinted with permission from Kendall CJ. *Ophthalmic Echography.* Thorofare, NJ: SLACK Incorporated; 1990.)

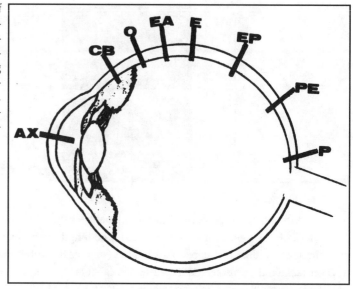

**Figure 5-18.** Just as in B-scan, the initial probe position for A-scan is the 6:00 limbus with the patient looking away, imaging the posterior portion of the 12:00 meridian, labeled 12:00 P. (Reprinted with permission from Kendall CJ. *Ophthalmic Echography.* Thorofare, NJ: SLACK Incorporated; 1990.)

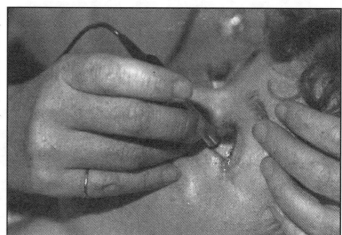

**Figure 5-19.** The probe is now halfway to the fornix, imaging the 12:00 meridian at about the equator of the globe, labeled 12:00 E. (Reprinted with permission from Kendall CJ. *Ophthalmic Echography.* Thorofare, NJ: SLACK Incorporated; 1990.)

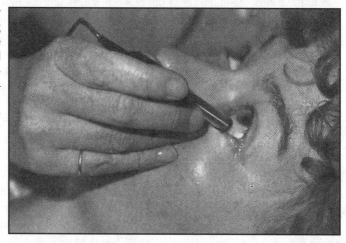

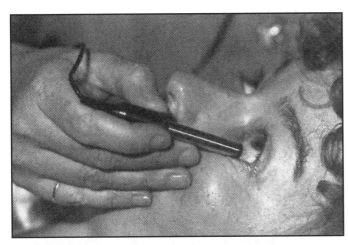

**Figure 5-20.** The probe is now at the fornix, imaging very anteriorly along the 12:00 meridian, labeled 12:00 CB for ciliary body. (Reprinted with permission from Kendall CJ. *Ophthalmic Echography.* Thorofare, NJ: SLACK Incorporated; 1990.)

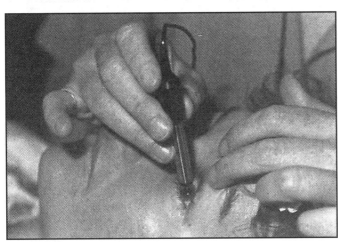

**Figure 5-21.** The 3:00 meridian is being examined posteriorly, 3:00 P. (Reprinted with permission from Kendall CJ. *Ophthalmic Echography.* Thorofare, NJ: SLACK Incorporated; 1990.)

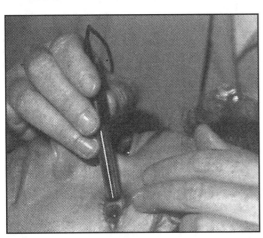

**Figure 5-22.** As the probe moves toward the inner canthus, the area being examined becomes 3:00 EP, between the equator and posterior pole. (Reprinted with permission from Kendall CJ. *Ophthalmic Echography.* Thorofare, NJ: SLACK Incorporated; 1990.)

**Figure 5-23.** The most extreme position of the probe now images 3:00 CB for ciliary body region. (Reprinted with permission from Kendall CJ. *Ophthalmic Echography.* Thorofare, NJ: SLACK Incorporated; 1990.)

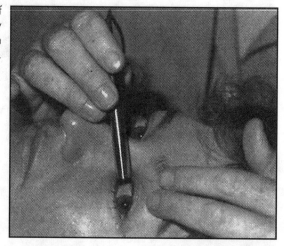

**Figure 5-24.** Screening of the superior globe (from posterior to anterior) using horizontal transverse approach. Note the probe marker is oriented nasally. (Reprinted with permission from Green RL, Bryne SF. Diagnostic ophthalmic ultrasound. In: Ryan SJ, ed. *Retina.* St. Louis, Mo: CV Mosby Co; 1989.)

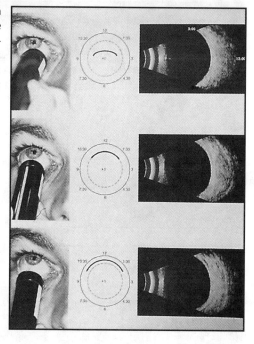

The B-scan screening procedure is first conducted with the instrument sensitivity placed at the high "tissue sensitivity" setting. This allows for detection of vitreous opacities and gross lesions. Then, the sensitivity is turned down in order to detect subtle (especially flat) lesions. The lower sensitivity improves tissue resolution.

In the event that a lesion is detected, the lesion must be assessed for size and position within the eye. This is done by using both A- and B-scan findings, and by comparing several B-scan views and putting the separate views together in one's mind. One of the most difficult aspects of B-scan ultrasonography is creating a three-dimensional image from several two-dimensional pictures. Let's say a lesion is detected in the 10:30 position while screening with the transverse approach. The transverse approach is re-evaluated by putting the probe on the 4:30 position (on the limbus) while the patient is looking up and to the right (in the 10:30 position). The probe marker is oriented 90 degrees away from 10:30, or in the superonasal position. The probe is moved from limbus to fornix as was previously described. This results in the sound beam being swept through the lesion from its most posterior to most anterior portion. This gives us information on the lesion's gross shape and dimension. Moreover, it provides information on the lesion's lateral extent, allowing the examiner to assess the lesion's gross width.

Once the location and the gross size has been estimated, a more exact measurement of the lesion must be made. This is done by using different probe positions to construct a three-dimensional picture from two-dimensional views. Next, the longitudinal view is scanned. In the longitudinal view the sound beam is oriented radially, with the beam perpendicular to the transverse view. When examining our theoretical lesion that has been located in the 10:30 meridian, the probe is placed on the limbus at 4:30, but this time the probe marker is oriented toward the cornea and the patient is looking in the 10:30 position. This gives us information on the anterior/posterior aspect of the lesion. (Remember, this view allows for the examination of the area between the optic nerve and the ora serrata.)

Finally, the lesion can be evaluated in relationship to other anatomical structures in the eye, namely the optic nerve and the lens. This is done using the axial view. When examining a lesion in the 10:30 position, the patient is instructed to look straight ahead. The probe is placed directly on the cornea with the marker oriented toward 10:30. With this probe orientation, the lesion will appear above the optic nerve on the display screen. By compiling the information obtained from these scans, we can create a three-dimensional image of the lesion.

## A- and B-Scan Used Together

Although the A-scan does not produce an image of the back of the eye, the information from the single dimension scan can be quite useful in the evaluation of masses, detachments, etc. After a mass has been detected and measured with B-scan ultrasonography, A-scan can be used to calculate size of the lesion, type of tissue involved, and/or kinetic response of the abnormality.

In the event that the ocular abnormality was a retinal detachment, the A-scan display may assist in the diagnosis. By looking at the spikes, we can determine the type of tissue involved. With a retinal detachment, there is a large spike, followed by a small flat section along the baseline, followed by another tall spike. This pattern indicates that the first tissue is highly reflective (as is the retina), and that there is a space between the retina and the sclera (as there is in a retinal detachment).

In the event that the abnormality is a tumor, the A-scan may reveal the type of internal structures that are present in the tumor. If the tissues are fairly similar throughout the tumor, there will be a large spike on the screen followed by a steep decline. In the event the tumor has many different types of cells, all of which have different sound velocities, there will be a large initial spike followed by multiple large spikes. Such differences can be quite useful in determining both the location of and the type of tissue present in an ocular mass.

Finally, we can evaluate kinetic aspects of lesions with both the A- and B-scans. The two types of motion that we might want to evaluate are mobility (or aftermovement), and vascularity (or spontaneous motion). Aftermovement represents mobility of the lesion after the eye has stopped moving. If there is movement in the echoes after the eye has stopped moving, this suggests that the lesion is not solid, such as a vitreous membrane or a retinal detachment. Such aftermovement of the echoes will not be produced by solid masses such as tumors. This differentiation can be important when conducting the examination. In order to evaluate aftermovement, the patient is asked to first fixate on a target while the lesion is viewed on the screen. The patient is then instructed to move the eye a short distance, and then back to the fixation target. Any movement of the lesion is noted by the echographer, who watches the image on the screen for the entire time. Any aftermovement is reported in the record.

Spontaneous movement of echoes while the eye is stationary suggests the presence of blood flow or vascularity. This is better evaluated with the A-scan, but can be detected on B-scan ultrasonography. In the event that a mass is expected to demonstrate blood flow, an A-scan should be performed. The patient is asked to remain perfectly still. The probe is placed so that its beam goes directly through the mass. The initial spike at the back of the eye represents the front part of the mass. If the spikes that follow the initial spike look blurred (presumably because of movement with the pulse), this suggests that there is active blood flow within the mass. With the B-scan, the examiner looks at the lesion to determine if spontaneous movement within the lesion can be detected. If movement can be reliably detected, one would suspect that the lesion is vascularized. Vascularity is a very important feature in the evaluation of mass-like lesions.

# Indications

Any time there is an inadequate view of the anterior or posterior segments, A- and B-scan ultrasonography may be indicated. First conduct both contact and non-contact B-scan ultrasonography (as well as diagnostic A-scan ultrasonography) in order to determine if the structures of the eye are normal. Systematically evaluate both the anterior and posterior chambers using the transverse and axial approaches. Also evaluate the iris, angle, lens, vitreous body, and the posterior aspect of the eye. If no lesions or abnormal echoes are detected, and the eye has been determined to be structurally normal, the examination is completed. However, if the examination reveals abnormality, then it becomes necessary to determine the exact structure involved and the extent of the abnormality. This is where aspects of topographic and kinetic ultrasonography are helpful. The remainder of this section will focus primarily on B-scan results. Keep in mind however, that an experienced ultrasonographer can easily use A-scan ultrasonography for such examinations.

## Disorders of the Vitreous

The most common indication for B-scan ultrasonography is vitreoretinal disease. The examiner may be looking for such things as vitreous opacities, vitreal detachments, retinal detachments, choroidal detachments, or scleral thickening. Therefore, the evaluation should include assessment of the following structures—vitreous body, posterior hyaloid, subvitreal space, retina, choroid, sclera, and optic disc.

The vitreous body should be evaluated first. The examiner should check the vitreous body for bands, opacities, and membranes. Vitreous opacities produce echoes that look like dots or small lines. Such opacities may consist of clumps of red blood cells, the cellular results of inflammation or infection, or calcium deposits. In the young normal eye, there should be no opacities present, thus the vitreous body should not produce echoes. In the normal aging eye there may be very low reflective opacities present in the vitreous. There may also be a posterior vitreous detachment present. These conditions generally do not represent pathology and are part of the natural changes that occur in the aging eye. Therefore, what might be considered abnormal in a young eye, would be considered normal in the eye of an older individual.

Vitreous hemorrhages may result from a number of conditions including trauma, diabetic retinopathy, age-related macular degeneration, retinal tears, and vein occlusions. B-scan ultrasonography is useful in establishing the density and location of the hemorrhage. In recent hemorrhages, the echoes may look like small dots or lines in the area of the hemorrhage. The more dense the hemorrhage, the greater the number of opacities that will be visible on the screen. In some cases of severe trauma, the vitreous may be virtually replaced by blood. This will result in significant opacities on the ultrasound.

Vitreous infection generally results from some type of surgical intervention or penetrating injury, although it is possible to develop endophthalmitis from a systemic process. The patient with endophthalmitis generally presents with signs of inflammation, pain, and inflammatory debris in the anterior chamber. B-scan will reveal diffuse, fine dot-like opacities in the vitreous. Also observable is diffuse thickening of the retino-choroid layer. Traction retinal detachments or serous retinal detachments may also be present. Inflammation such as uveitis has similar ultrasonographic findings. Therefore, it is essential that a thorough history be taken on each patient who has an ultrasound examination.

Calcium deposits may also be present in the vitreous, resulting in observable opacities on ultrasonography. These calcium soaps produce bright, point-like echoes on the B-scan. These opacities may be diffuse or localized within the vitreous. This pattern is associated with asteroid hyalosis (Figure 5-25).

### Vitreous Detachment

A posterior vitreous detachment may be a common finding in older patients, as indicated above. The detachment may be either localized or extensive. The hyaloid may be completely separated from the optic nerve head, or may attach at the nerve head. If there is complete detachment, including the optic nerve, then the detachment is of the vitreous and not the retina. (In a complete retinal detachment, there is always an insertion point at the optic nerve.) If there is an attachment at the optic nerve, then it becomes necessary to differentiate between a possible vitreous versus retinal detachment.

In B-scan ultrasonography, there is a reflective line (posterior vitreous face) along the area of detachment. If the detachment is actually a vitreous detachment and not a retinal detachment then the line will be fine, and will appear quite mobile on kinetic B-scan ultrasonography (Figure 5-26). If the detachment is a retinal detachment, then the line will appear thicker, and will not be too mobile on kinetic B-scan ultrasonography. The presence of good mobility and the thin, linear echo generally assures the examiner that the echo represents a vitreous detachment and not a retinal detachment.

## Disorders of the Retina

One of the most important aspects of B-scan ultrasonography is its role in evaluating the retina of patients with opaque media. Certainly one of the first questions asked by the referring physician is whether the retina is attached or detached. In the event that the retina is detached, the ultrasonographer can locate the detachment and estimate its extent (partial, complete, tear, etc).

A thorough evaluation of the quadrants of the eye may allow for the detection of even the smallest retinal tears. The tears are frequently found in the superior peripheral fundus. In many instances, a vitreous detachment or vitreous strand is attached to the tear.

Retinal detachments generally produce a bright echo that appears to be continuous. There may be some folds present and there is generally an insertion at the optic nerve head. If the detachment is either extensive or total, there are two places of insertion—the optic nerve and the ora serrata. The detached retina is somewhat mobile, but far less mobile than a total vitreous detachment. A total retinal detachment may be funnel shaped, triangular shaped, or (if the retina has been detached for an extensive amount of time) T-shaped (Figures 5-27 thorough 5-29).

**Figure 5-25.** A patient with asteroid hyalosis has calcium deposits in the vitreous (AH). The asteroid bodies are clearly visible even with reduced gain, due to their highly reflective nature. (Reprinted with permission from Kendall CJ. *Ophthalmic Echography.* Thorofare, NJ: SLACK Incorporated; 1990.)

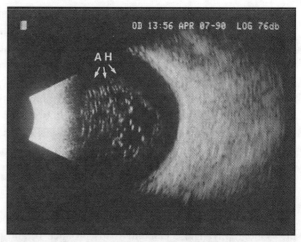

**Figure 5-26.** Classic case of a traction retinal detachment. Vitreous membrane (VM) has contracted pulling off the retina (R). The point of attachment between the two membranes is shown with the center arrow. Note the fine line of the vitreous echo, as opposed to the thicker line of the retina echo. (Reprinted with permission from Kendall CJ. *Ophthalmic Echography.* Thorofare, NJ: SLACK Incorporated; 1990.)

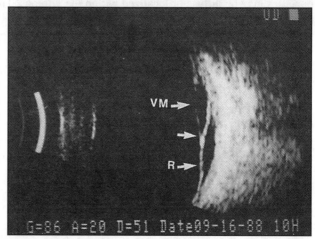

**Figure 5-27.** Axial B-scan of an open funnel-shaped retinal detachment. (Reprinted with permission from Green RL, Bryne SF. Diagnostic ophthalmic ultrasound. In: Ryan SJ, ed. *Retina.* St. Louis, Mo: CV Mosby Co; 1989.)

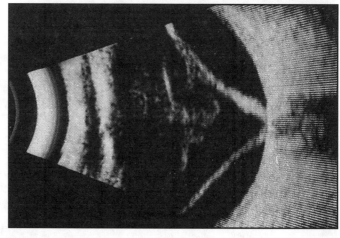

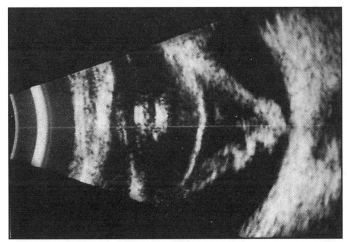

**Figure 5-28.** Axial B-scan of a triangular funnel-shaped retinal detachment. (Reprinted with permission from Green RL, Bryne SF. Diagnostic ophthalmic ultrasound. In: Ryan SJ, ed. *Retina.* St. Louis, Mo: CV Mosby Co; 1989.)

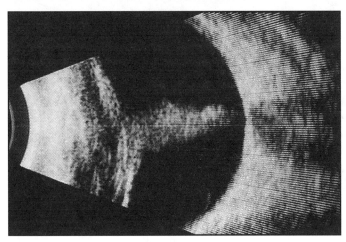

**Figure 5-29.** Axial B-scan of a "T" funnel-shaped (closed funnel) retinal detachment. (Reprinted with permission from Green RL, Bryne SF. Diagnostic ophthalmic ultrasound. In: Ryan SJ, ed. *Retina.* St. Louis, Mo: CV Mosby Co; 1989.)

## Disorders of the Choroid

### Thickening

Choroidal thickening can be detected on B-scan ultrasonography. This condition may be associated with many ocular disorders. Thickening of the choroid may be localized or diffuse, and appears as a widened area on the scan while viewing the posterior portion of the eye. The reflectivity of the choroid may be high or low, and this relative reflectivity may be associated with certain ocular conditions. Choroidal thickening that is highly reflective is often associated with such disorders as choroidal edema, hypotony, endophthalmitis, and uveitis. Choroidal thickening that is low in reflectivity may be associated with such conditions as Vogt-Koyanagi-Harada syndrome or sympathetic ophthalmia.

### Detachment

Choroidal detachment is often associated with trauma or surgical intervention, but can occur spontaneously. Choroidal detachments produce characteristic echographic findings, so differentiation is generally quite easy. Choroidal detachments usually look like smooth, dome-shaped membranes. They are often located in the periphery, and on occasion are detached for 360 degrees.

When this occurs, they produce scalloped-edged membranes (Figure 5-30). If the membranes touch, they are referred to as kissing choroidals (Figure 5-31).

## Disorders of the Optic Nerve

There are some instances where B-scan ultrasonography is useful in assessing the optic nerve head and the retrobulbar area of the optic nerve. Optic nerve colobomas, as well as large optic cups, can be detected with the B-scan. Optic nerve drusen appear as highly reflective nodules overlying the optic nerve when viewed with the B-scan (Figure 5-32). Retrobulbar optic nerve disease can also be assessed using the B-scan. The normal optic nerve produces a characteristic pattern that looks like a narrow, black "V" extending from the back of the eye. When there is enlargement of the retrobulbar optic nerve, this "V" shape increases in width. The presence or absence of optic nerve thickening can be determined using both B-scan and A-scan ultrasonography.

## Intraocular Tumors

Diagnostic B-scan ultrasonography is an essential tool used to detect, differentiate, measure, and follow intraocular tumors. Standardized Echography provides accurate measurement of tumor height and locality. It is beyond the scope of this book to detail ultrasonographic findings in each tumor type; however, a brief description of two types of important tumors will be presented.

### Ocular Melanoma

Ocular melanoma is a potentially life-threatening malignant tumor of the eye. It is similar to other types of melanoma and can be located in several structures within the eye including the iris, the ciliary body, and the choroid. Several key characteristics are present in most ocular melanomas, allowing for accurate diagnosis. Those characteristics include mushroom or collar-button shape on B-scan, solid consistency, internal vascularity, regular internal structure, and low to medium reflectivity of the B-scan echoes. Echography can also be useful after treatment to determine if the tumor has shrunk or not (Figure 5-33 through 5-35).

### Retinoblastomas

Retinoblastomas are another type of potentially life-threatening tumor seen in young children that can be diagnosed using Standardized Echography. The determination that a tumor is a retinoblastoma is frequently based on the echographic finding of calcium within the tumor. Calcium is highly reflective, and calcium deposits within a childhood intraocular tumor is highly suggestive of retinoblastoma. Calcification may be minimal or very abundant. Retinoblastomas may present as large masses located either posterior or anterior to the retina. They may also appear as diffuse lesions at the retina. They may be bumpy or irregular in appearance. Intraocular tumors that have these characteristics should be considered suspicious for retinoblastoma. Ultrasonography may be helpful in the follow-up phase after treatment to determine if the tumor's size has been reduced.

## Trauma

B-scan ultrasonography can be useful in many cases involving trauma. Ultrasonography can detect the presence of wounds, vitreous hemorrhages, retinal detachments, and choroidal detachments, as well as evaluate the general shape of the eye. Ultrasonography can be useful in the pre-operative evaluation of a traumatized eye. If the eye is completely disorganized, then the physician may opt to remove the eye instead of repair it.

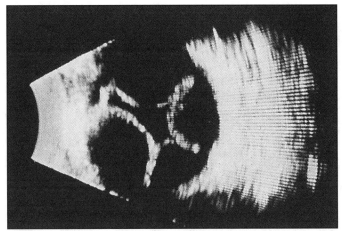

**Figure 5-30.** Extremely peripheral transverse section through 360-degree choroidal detachment shows classic scalloped shape. (Reprinted with permission from Green RL, Bryne SF. Diagnostic ophthalmic ultrasound. In: Ryan SJ, ed. *Retina.* St. Louis, Mo: CV Mosby Co; 1989.)

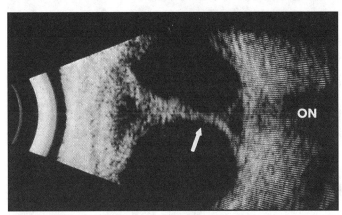

**Figure 5-31.** Axial view of choroidal detachment showing typical kissing choroidal appearance. *ON*, optic nerve. (Reprinted with permission from Green RL, Bryne SF. Diagnostic ophthalmic ultrasound. In: Ryan SJ, ed. *Retina.* St. Louis, Mo: CV Mosby Co; 1989.)

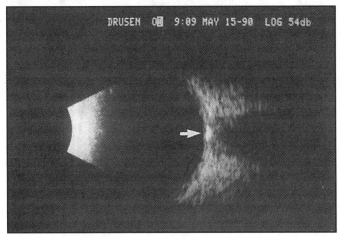

**Figure 5-32.** Disk drusen is a calcium deposit on the optic nerve head. This calcium is so different from ocular tissue that it appears as a foreign body, a bright echo even when the gain is turned way down. The optic nerve shadow is often wider in these cases. (Reprinted with permission from Kendall CJ. *Ophthalmic Echography.* Thorofare, NJ: SLACK Incorporated; 1990.)

**Figure 5-33.** A malignant melanoma of the choroid that is classified as small in size. (Reprinted with permission from Kendall CJ. *Ophthalmic Echography.* Thorofare, NJ: SLACK Incorporated; 1990.)

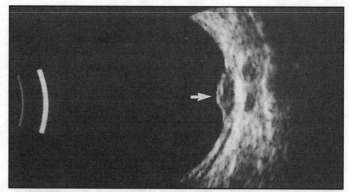

**Figure 5-34.** A malignant melanoma of the choroid that is classified as medium in size. (Reprinted with permission from Kendall CJ. *Ophthalmic Echography.* Thorofare, NJ: SLACK Incorporated; 1990.)

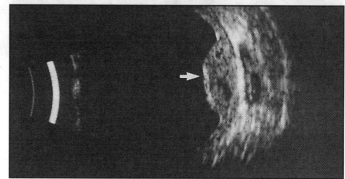

**Figure 5-35.** A malignant melanoma of the choroid that is classified as large in size. (Reprinted with permission from Kendall CJ. *Ophthalmic Echography.* Thorofare, NJ: SLACK Incorporated; 1990.)

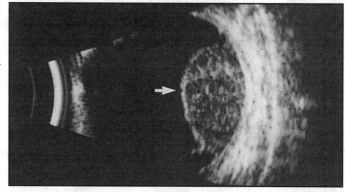

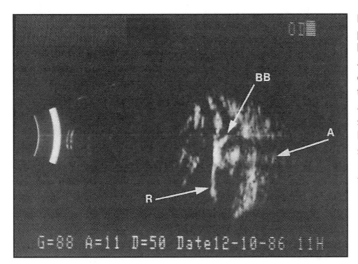

**Figure 5-36.** A steel BB from a pellet gun has an unmistakable bright echo from the surface, and a chain of reverberation echoes that follow. In this case, the BB is under the retina (R), and the artifact echoes (A) are seen posterior to the foreign body. (Reprinted with permission from Kendall CJ. *Ophthalmic Echography.* Thorofare, NJ: SLACK Incorporated; 1990.)

Frequently, individuals who have experienced a penetrating injury to the eye have retained foreign bodies. B-scan ultrasonography can be helpful in detecting such material (Figure 5-36). It has been suggested that B-scan ultrasonography be obtained even when an intraocular foreign body has been detected on CT scan. This is because ocular ultrasonography is more precise in localizing the foreign body. B-scan ultrasonography can establish whether the foreign body is just inside or just outside the eye. Finally, ultrasonography can be helpful in determining the type of foreign body that is present. Generally, metallic foreign bodies are irregular in shape and are highly reflective, thus producing very strong echoes even when the sensitivity is low. Moreover, there is usually a dark shadow behind the metallic foreign body because the metal reflects virtually everything back to the probe. Extremely small metallic foreign bodies will behave similarly to larger foreign bodies, but the shadowing will not be as marked.

Glass foreign bodies are frequently difficult to detect, so it is essential that a thorough examination be conducted when retained glass is suspected. Glass generally enters the eye as a sliver-shaped shard. When the sound beams from the probe hit the long portion of the sliver in a nonperpendicular manner (that is, head-on), there will be very little echo reflected back to the probe. It is not until the sound beam hits the glass perpendicularly (from the side) that a highly reflective object can be detected. This pattern is suggestive of a glass foreign body.

Wood and other vegetable-type foreign bodies may produce varying ultrasonographic findings. Initially the foreign body may be highly reflective. As the organic substance starts to decompose its reflectivity will decrease. This dynamic presentation can be indicative of the presence of wood or other vegetable-matter foreign bodies.

# Reference

1. Ossoinig KC. Standardized echography: basic principles, clinical applications and results. *Int Ophthalmol Clin.* 1979:127-210.

# Part III

# Electrophysiology Testing

# Introduction to Ocular Electrophysiology

Ocular electrophysiology is similar to other types of electrophysiologic tests that you may have heard of during your healthcare career. Generally speaking, electrophysiologic tests are conducted to determine how well some portion of the body is functioning. The test that you might be most familiar with is the electrocardiogram (EKG). When an EKG is ordered, the cardiologist is trying to determine if the electrical activity of the heart is normal. The cardiologist will look for specific patterns in the EKG tracing to determine if the heart is functioning abnormally or normally. If the waveform is abnormal, the cardiologist will be able to determine what type of abnormality is present and in which area of the heart the abnormality is located.

In the case of ocular electrophysiology, the eyecare specialist is trying to determine how well the visual system is working. The ophthalmologist may be interested in the electrical activity of the retina or how well the optic nerve and visual cortex are working. Ocular electrophysiology provides those answers.

There are three main tests that will be covered in this section on ocular electrophysiology. They include the electroretinogram (ERG), the electro-oculogram (EOG), and the visual evoked response (VER; sometimes called the visual evoked potential or VEP). Ocular electrophysiology tests are used much less than many of the other types of electrophysiologic tests that are available. Do not be surprised if you do not know much about these tests. They are performed on very few patients and are almost always performed in large university settings. The tests must be conducted using special computerized equipment and should be administered only by highly trained specialists.

Electrophysiology tests are diagnostic in nature, and are objective. You may ask a patient what he or she can read on an eye chart. If the patient is not very cooperative, he or she may not answer you. If the person is malingering, he or she might tell you that only the fingers on your hand are visible, while possessing 20/20 vision. In ocular electrophysiology, the tests require no response from the patient. The patient cannot fake the results of the tests since the patient cannot control his or her electrical responses to the stimuli that are presented during the tests. The tests do require some cooperation from the patient, but can be performed on virtually anyone (generally speaking).

## Brief History

Electrophysiologic testing has been around, in at least a rudimentary form, since the 18th century (Table III-1). Galvani discovered in the 1700s that nerve cells had electricity. From that point forward there have been significant advances in the field of electrophysiology. In 1849 DuBois discovered an electrical potential difference between the front and the back of the eye; in 1865 Holmgren performed the first animal ERG. In 1877 Dewar conducted the first ERG and EOG on humans. Between 1950 and 1970 significant information was obtained on human ERGs and EOGs, thus supporting their usefulness in detecting certain ocular conditions. The first VER in humans was conducted by Cruikshank in 1937. Due to the nature of the VER, a useful technique was not perfected until the advent of computers. In 1954 Dawson conducted the first VER to use a summated approach that was able to differentiate small visual potentials from large resting brain activity. By 1963, VERs were used clinically.

Ocular electrophysiology has become an important aspect of clinical ophthalmology over the years. Each test will be reviewed so that its usefulness in an eyecare setting can be better understood.

Table III-1.
# Electrophysiology Tests Throughout History

| | EOG | ERG | VER |
|---|---|---|---|
| 1849 | DuBois—Raymond observed an electric potential difference between the front and the back of the eye | | |
| 1865 | | Holmgren—retinal-electrical recordings in fish | |
| 1877 | | Dewar—1st humans | |
| 1927 | | | Adrian—discharge in the optic nerve comes from retinal electric change |
| 1933 | | Granit—cat retina rods have A, B, and C waves | Gerard—animals, occipital recordings respond to light |
| 1936 | Mowrer—retinal origin in cats | | |
| 1937 | | | Cruikshank—1st VER humans |
| 1941 | | Riggs—human contact lens electrode | |
| 1945 | | Karpe—clinical study of 64 normal, 87 abnormal patients | |
| 1952 | | Cobb—bright flash testing | |
| 1953 | Noell—EOG arises from RPE function in rabbits | | |
| 1954 | | Riggs—abnormal ERG in right-blind humans (RP) | Dawson—VER summation technique helps see small potential |
| 1956 | Francois—human retinal diseases | | |
| 1962 | Arden—max. in light adapt, min. in dark adapt, pigmentary degenerations | | |
| 1963 | | | Copenhaven—VER clinical studies begin |
| 1966 | Krill et al.—Best's vitelliform maculopathy | | |
| 1967 | Klien and Krill—fundus flavimaculata | | |
| 1972 | | | Halliday—VER prolonged in optic neuritis |

*(Reprinted with permission from Benes SC, McKinney K, Sanders LC, Miller M, Moberg M.* Advanced Ophthalmic Diagnostics and Therapeutics. *SLACK Incorporated, 1990.)*

Chapter 6

# Electroretinography

KEY POINTS

- The electroretinogram (ERG) is an objective test of retinal function.

- The ERG records a mass retinal response, so individuals with focal retinal pathology will have normal ERG findings.

- The testing parameters can be modified so that either cone, rod, or cone and rod photoreceptor cells can be tested.

- The test requires some cooperation on the part of the patient, so it may not be suitable for infants or young children who are not sedated.

# Introduction to the Electroretinogram

The full-field electroretinogram (ERG) is an electrical response or action potential of the retina to a brief flash of light. The ERG is a test of the entire retinal area and is used to evaluate both cone and rod photoreceptor cell activity. In order to record an ERG, a light is flashed into the patient's eyes. This causes all of the photoreceptor cells within the retina to fire simultaneously (referred to as a mass retinal response). This mass response results in a waveform that is detected by means of a corneal contact lens electrode (worn by the patient). The ERG waveform represents both photoreceptor, Müller and bi-polar cell activity. The photoreceptor, Müller, and bi-polar cells are positioned radially within the eye. Due to this positioning, the electrical currents from these cells flow easily through the vitreous and cornea, thus allowing for detection of these small electrical responses by means of corneal electrodes. The electrode is connected to a computer and the response is displayed on the computer's monitor. (Generally the corneal electrode is used, but other types are available.) The ERG is an excellent test to determine how well the entire retina is functioning.

There are two other types of ERGs that can be recorded. One type is referred to as the focal or macular electroretinogram (MERG), while the other is known as the pattern electroretinogram (PERG).

The MERG tests a very small patch of retina, generally the macula. Instead of using a flashing light that illuminates the entire retina, a small focal light (usually attached to a modified direct ophthalmoscope) is used to stimulate a small part of the retina. This test is frequently used to evaluate macular function or macular pathology, but can be used to test other focal areas of the retina.

The PERG is used to test ganglion cell function. An alternating checkerboard pattern is illuminated on the retina. The patient must be able to see the alternating checkerboard pattern clearly, so electrodes that do not cover the cornea are frequently used. The illumination of the alternating pattern on the retina results in cone stimulation, but the waveform represents ganglion cell activity. The ganglion cell response is then detected at the front of the eye by the electrode.

The type of ERG recorded (either full-field, focal, or pattern) will result in different types of electrical activity being generated by the retina. Consequently, the waveforms being recorded at the cornea will also look different from one another.

Clinical practices rely almost exclusively on full-field ERG testing to detect retinal pathology. As this is the most clinically significant of the ERGs, the remainder of the chapter will be dedicated to describing this test.

## Understanding Photoreceptor Cell Function

In order to better understand the components of the ERG and the significance of the testing parameters that will be described, a brief review of photoreceptor cell function will be presented.

Humans have very complex visual systems that allow us to see fairly well in both daytime and nighttime conditions. This is due to the fact that there are two types of photoreceptors within the eye—the cones and the rods. The cones provide fine, detailed vision and color perception. The cones do not function well in the dark and are sensitive only to bright lights. In other words, cones provide us with our daytime vision. Rods, on the other hand, do not function well in the daytime. They do not perceive color, and do not see fine detail. The primary function of the rods is to see in the dark. In other words, rods provide us with our nighttime vision.

Although rods function best in the dark, it takes them about 30 minutes in order to be nearly fully dark-adapted. It also takes the rods a few minutes to "figure out" that they are in the dark. Think of a time when you were suddenly in total darkness and how poorly you were able to see for the first couple of minutes. That is because your cones were still functioning and were not doing a very good job of seeing in the dark. After about 5 minutes your vision should have been much better, and you should have been able to see some objects. The rods were starting to work. They were not working near to their fullest potential until you had been in the dark for another 30 minutes or so. No matter how long you stay in the dark, your visual acuity and your detail vision will never improve. Only your ability to see dimmer and dimmer lights will improve. After being in the dark for 30 minutes, an individual is able to see about 100,000 times better than he or she did when first put in the dark (see Chapter 2, Dark Adaptometry Testing).

In the clinical setting, you may have patients tell you that they do not see well in the dark. Individuals may report that things appear "grainy" or "fuzzy." That is perfectly normal. A patient may report that he or she cannot differentiate colors or read in the dark. That, too, is perfectly normal since rods do not provide color or central vision. If a patient reports being unable to see "anything in the dark," the person may truly have nyctalopia (night blindness). An easy way to determine if a person has nyctalopia is to turn off all the lights in the examination room. (You must stay in the room with the patient.) After 5 minutes, ask the patient to identify objects in the room. If the patient cannot see things that you can see easily (assuming that you have normal rod function) the patient may truly have retinal problems affecting the rods.

Understanding rod and cone function is very important in the study of the ERG. Examiners can manipulate the testing environment in order to test only rods, only cones, or both rods and cones simultaneously.

# The Full-Field ERG

The full-field ERG is a useful test to determine how well an individual's retina is functioning. This may be helpful in providing a diagnosis for the patient or in providing prognostic information about the patient's retinal condition. During ERG testing, a light of specific intensity is flashed into the patient's eyes, resulting in the sudden illumination of the retina. When the retina is suddenly illuminated, all of the cells within the illuminated area are activated simultaneously, resulting in a particular type of waveform. (The shape of the waveform is dependent on which type of photoreceptor cells are stimulated.)

It is only possible to stimulate the entire retina if a technique known as full-field or Ganzfeld stimulation is used, which results in a mass retinal response. Full-field or Ganzfeld stimulation is achieved by having the patient tested within a Ganzfeld bowl (similar to a perimeter) (Figure 6-1). A frosted contact lens electrode can also be used for retinal stimulation, but is not recommended by authorities in ocular electrophysiology.[1]

The Ganzfeld bowl (or frosted contact lens) results in the light entering the eye in a diffused manner. As a result, instead of illuminating the retina only in the area of the posterior pole, the light is scattered and illuminates the entire retinal area (Figure 6-2). When Ganzfeld stimulation is used, the amplitude of the response corresponds to how much of the retina is working. If, for instance, a patient has a 50% retinal detachment, then the ERG in the affected eye will be reduced in amplitude by 50% as compared with the normal fellow eye. If a person has a 25% retinal detachment, the ERG will be reduced by 25%, and so forth. This rule applies in most, but not all instances. If a small area of retina is damaged (the macula for example), then the ERG will be reduced by a small amount (less than 1%). However, the reduction may be difficult to detect because small differences of up to 10% between the two eyes are normal.

Conversely, if only a small area of retina is working, again let's say the macula, then the ERG may be so small as to be undetectable at the cornea by many commercially available electro-

**Figure 6-1.** The inside of the brightly lit hemispheric Ganzfeld bowl, with the chin rest centered. (Reprinted with permission from Benes SC, McKinney K, Sanders LC, Miller M, Moberg M. *Advanced Ophthalmic Diagnostics and Therapeutics.* Thorofare, NJ: SLACK Incorporated; 1990.)

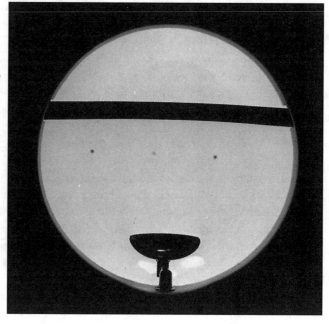

**Figure 6-2.** The entire back of the retina is stimulated by means of light scattering when a Ganzfeld bowl is used. This can also be done by using a frosted contact lens on the eye, as shown here. (Reprinted with permission from Carr RE, Siegel IM. *Electrodiagnostic Testing of the Visual System: A Clinical Guide.* Philadelphia, Pa: FA Davis Co; 1990.)

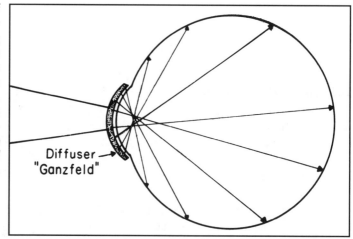

physiology units. This will result in a non-recordable ERG. As a result, an ERG can be normal in a person with very poor acuity, or non-recordable in a person with fairly good acuity. This brings us to another important point to remember about the standard ERG—there is not a direct correlation between ERGs and visual acuity.

## Materials Needed for Recording the ERG

In order to perform an ERG (or any of the other ocular electrophysiology tests mentioned in this book) one must have access to an ocular electrodiagnostic unit. A unit generally comes equipped with a computer, a signal averager, a pre-amplifier (into which the electrodes are plugged), a monitor, a Ganzfeld bowl with stimulator, and a printer (Figure 6-3).

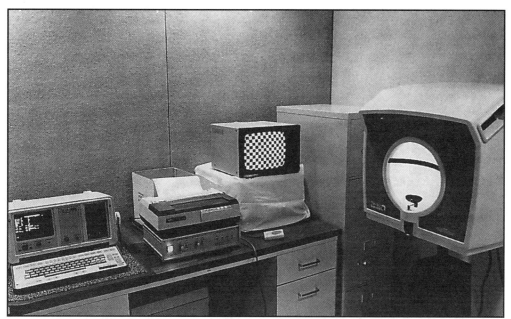

**Figure 6-3.** An electrodiagnostic unit with (from right to left) a Ganzfeld bowl, checkerboard monitor, printer, and computer with screen. (Reprinted with permission from Benes SC, McKinney K, Sanders LC, Miller M, Moberg M. *Advanced Ophthalmic Diagnostics and Therapeutics.* Thorofare, NJ: SLACK Incorporated; 1990.)

this book) one must have access to an ocular electrodiagnostic unit. A unit generally comes equipped with a computer, a signal averager, a pre-amplifier (into which the electrodes are plugged), a monitor, a Ganzfeld bowl with stimulator, and a printer (Figure 6-3).

## Electrodes

Two types of electrodes are used for recording the ERG. The first is an active electrode. This is generally a corneal electrode that rests on the eye, either directly on or adjacent to the cornea. This active electrode comes in several varieties. There are contact lens-type electrodes as well as electrodes made of electro-conductive materials such as gold foil, silver carpet fiber, or coated copper wire (there are little slits in the plastic coating) (Figure 6-4). The active electrodes are either bipolar or monopolar. The bipolar electrode contains both an active and reference electrode. Burian-Allen (Hansen Ophthalmic Development Laboratory, Iowa City, Iowa) contact lens electrodes are usually bipolar, but can also be monopolar. The monopolar electrode contains only an active electrode.

The second type of electrode is the reference electrode. This electrode is either a gold or silver chloride cup electrode that is placed on the skin. If the active electrode is monopolar, such as the gold foil, Jet (The Electrode Store, Enumclaws, Wash.) contact lens, or carpet fiber electrodes, then a reference electrode must be placed on the patients face. The reference electrode is placed either at the lateral canthus or on the forehead slightly above the eyebrow and directly over the eye.

A ground electrode is also used in ERG testing. This electrode does not record ERG activity, but helps stabilize the waveform, resulting in better ERG recordings. The ground electrode is

**Figure 6-4.** Three types of electrodes used for ERG testing. (Photograph by Nilo Davila.)

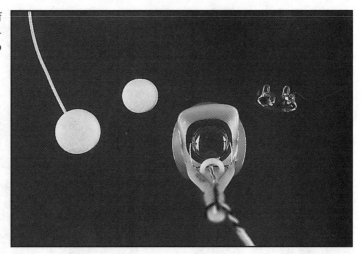

### Electrode Selection

In most instances, the best type of electrode to use for standard ERG testing is the Burian-Allen contact lens-style electrode. The active electrode of this contact lens rests directly over the cornea, thus allowing for the most direct recording of retinal activity. (The farther away the electrode is from the cornea, the smaller the response.) This electrode also has a speculum attached to it, which keeps the eye open during testing. This allows for the greatest amount of retinal stimulation to occur. However, this electrode is very uncomfortable for some, especially those who have sustained recent ocular trauma. This electrode comes in a wide variety of sizes to accommodate eyes of adults, children, and very small infants.

The Jet electrode is a contact lens electrode that rests on the cornea (thus having some of the advantages of the Burian-Allen style), but it does not have a speculum. There are small posts on the anterior surface of the lens and the patient can close his or her eyes over the posts. This can be very painful. This electrode style is only good for individuals who are very cooperative. The lenses are disposable and fairly inexpensive, making them useful when disposability is required (such as when the patient is suspected of having EKC).

The carpet fiber, gold foil, and wire loop electrodes are excellent for recording responses in people who have some mild corneal problems. Most of these electrodes are designed to be disposable, although the wire loop is a multi-use electrode. They are designed to rest in the lower cul-de-sac, which makes them more comfortable. These types of electrodes are ideal for recording pattern ERGs, where the patient must be able to view the television pattern clearly. They can be used successfully with young children and infants (especially the wire loop electrode).

Individuals who are fearful of having their eyes touched may find this test more uncomfortable. Using a smaller Burian-Allen contact lens electrode or using a fiber electrode may be better for this type of patient. Do not use a Jet electrode on someone who is nervous about having his or her eyes touched, as this electrode is sometimes difficult to remove.

In some instances a patient will be unable to tolerate any electrode on the eye (usually as a result of trauma or due to a very compromised cornea). When this occurs, two skin electrodes can be used to record an ERG. One serves as the active electrode and the other as the reference electrode. In such instances, the skin electrodes are placed under the eye (active position) and on the forehead above the eye (reference position), with the ground electrode on the forehead in the midline position.

## What the Patient Needs to Know

- (When the test is scheduled) Your eyes will be dilated and there will be some blurring after the test. You will probably need someone to drive you home.

- Do not wear eye makeup, or be prepared to remove eye makeup if you wear it to the appointment. Makeup can get into the eyes during the ERG and cause irritation.

- (The day of the test) The test is not painful, but may be somewhat uncomfortable. A numbing drop will be used.

- Do not squeeze the eye, as this will increase the discomfort while the lens is being inserted.

- Try not to move or blink your eyes during the test. Such movement will make recording the ERG much more difficult.

- In rare cases, some people notice a headache after the test. Take a regular pain reliever if the headache persists.

- If you have epilepsy, please tell us.

- After the test, do not to touch or rub your eyes, since the eyes may remain numb for several minutes after the test.

- Your vision will remain blurry for the next hour or so as a result of the procedure. This is normal.

- Your eyes may feel a little uncomfortable for several hours after the test, but should not be painful.

- See your ophthalmologist if the eye becomes red or excessively painful.

Any of these electrodes will record an ERG. Each type has its advantages and its disadvantages. The contact lens variety will produce the largest ERG, yet may be uncomfortable for the patient. The carpet fiber, gold foil, and wire loops may be better tolerated, but may produce smaller waveforms. The disposable electrodes will insure that disease is not spread between patients, yet some can be very expensive. The skin electrodes will be tolerated best, but will produce very small and often unreliable responses. Test results can be negatively affected by distance of the electrodes from the cornea, facial movement by the patient, or moisture coming from the skin or eyes. Regardless of the type of electrode used, ERG detection will be similar.

### Other Materials

Several eye drops must be used for the ERG (Figure 6-5). Regardless of the type of ERG recorded, the patient's pupils must be dilated. This allows adequate retinal illumination during testing. Since most of the active electrodes rest on the patient's eyes, it is essential that the eyes be adequately anesthetized during testing. A commercially available topical anesthetic can be used. The corneal contact lens electrode must be covered with a methylcellulose solution of at least 1.0% in order to keep the cornea moist during testing. Finally, a conductive electrode paste must be used with the skin electrodes, which are attached to the skin with surgical tape. Some skin electrodes come with self-adhesive attachments that contain the conductive electrode paste.

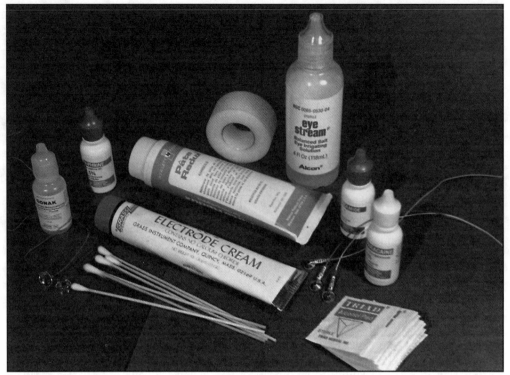

**Figure 6-5.** Materials needed for ERG testing. (Reprinted with permission from Benes SC, McKinney K, Sanders LC, Miller M, Moberg M. *Advanced Ophthalmic Diagnostics and Therapeutics.* Thorofare, NJ: SLACK Incorporated; 1990.)

## Recording a Full-Field ERG According to International Standards

Back in 1989, the International Society for the Clinical Electrophysiology of Vision and the National Retinitis Pigmentosa Foundation, Inc., developed a committee to establish international standards for ERG testing. These standards were developed so that all ERGs would be recorded in a similar manner. The aim was to make sure that ERGs were equivalent between laboratories and within research publications. Before the standards were established, many laboratories had their "own way" of recording ERGs, thus making it impossible for others to interpret the data. The standards have all but eliminated these problems. Individual laboratories can still have their own way of doing ERG recordings, but the means by which the ERG is recorded must be shown to be comparable to international standards if any of the data from the laboratory is to be published. Also, individual laboratories can customize certain aspects of the ERG test, but need to include at least the waveforms listed in the sections on recording dark-adapted and light-adapted ERGs.

### Patient Set-up

Prior to recording the ERG, the patient's eye should be viewed with a direct ophthalmoscope to see if the eye is quiet. If the eye does not appear quiet, then a slit lamp examination should follow and the abnormality noted. Patients with conjunctivitis, recent trauma, recent surgical wounds, or compromised corneas (ulcers, lacerations, etc) should not be tested by means of corneal electrodes. In these cases, consult with the doctor and determine if the test should be deferred.

After the patient's eyes have been evaluated, test the visual acuity and note it in the chart. The patient should then be informed of the procedure. Next, the patient should be dilated with phenylephrine 2.5% and tropicamide 1%. While the patient is dilating, he or she should also be dark-adapting for at least 20 minutes. Dark adaptation can be done in the ERG examining room with the room lights off (providing there are no light leaks) or by having the patient wear a pair of red goggles that cover the eyes entirely. The red goggles dark-adapt the eyes while allowing the patient to remain in the waiting room.

Once the patient has been dark-adapted for 20 to 30 minutes, the ERG can take place. Make sure the patient does not become light-adapted when you come into or leave the examining room. Putting a sign on the examining room door can be helpful, to assure that no one walks into the darkened examining room during scotopic testing.

The room in which the ERG is performed should have a red light, like a photographic dark-room. This allows you and the patient to see without ruining the patient's dark-adapted state. Position the patient in front of the Ganzfeld bowl and adjust the position of the chair so that the person can comfortably put his or her chin on the chin rest. Some patients cannot tolerate sitting erect and therefore must lie down during the ERG. The Ganzfeld bowl can be attached to an apparatus that suspends it, thus allowing it to be swiveled to any position over a patient's face.

Next, determine what type of active electrode is going to be needed for the procedure. If a bipolar electrode is going to be used, prepare the skin for the ground electrode. Scrub a small area of the forehead in the midline position with a skin cleaner; 70% isopropyl alcohol or a skin prep solution such as Omni-Prep (DO Weaver and Co, Aurora, Colo) are excellent choices. Next, fill the skin electrode with electrode conduction paste such as EC-2 Electrode Cream (Grass Instruments Company, Quincy, Mass.) and place it on the cleansed area of skin. Cover the electrode with surgical tape to insure good contact throughout the test. The ground electrode can also be placed behind one ear. Attach the electrode in a manner similar to that described above.

Anesthetize the eye with a topical anesthetic. If the patient is going to wear a contact lens electrode, fill the contact lens with 1 or 2.5% methylcellulose so that the cornea is protected during the test. Remind the patient not to squeeze the eye, as this will result in discomfort during insertion of the contact lens electrode.

If the active electrode is a Burian-Allen type of contact lens that has a speculum attached to it, have the patient look down and slip the upper speculum under the upper lid. Then ask the patient to look up and slip the lower speculum under the lower lid. If the active electrode is a Jet contact lens electrode or one of the other monopolar conductive material electrodes, place a reference electrode above each eye using a similar procedure as that used for the ground electrode. (The patient will then have three skin electrodes on the face—one on the forehead and one above each eye.) The reference electrode can also be placed below and temporal to the eye.

If the patient is going to wear the Jet contact lens electrode, ask him or her to look straight ahead while you pull the lids apart slightly with one hand. With the other hand, put the contact lens directly on the cornea. Again, remind the patient not to squeeze the eye, as the lids may be able to go over the little pegs that are on the outside of this electrode. (They are designed to keep the eye open during testing.) (See Figures 6-6 through 6-13.)

If a gold foil or silver carpet fiber electrode is used, have the patient look up slightly while gently pulling down on the lower lid. The electrode is then placed in the lower cul-de-sac and the wire attached to the electrode is secured onto the patient's lower lid with tape to reduce slippage during testing.

**Figure 6-6.** The area of the skin where the reference electrode is placed should be prepped with alcohol. Reference electrodes are needed when monopolar electrodes, such as the Jet, are used. (Reprinted with permission from Benes SC, McKinney K, Sanders LC, Miller M, Moberg M. *Advanced Ophthalmic Diagnostics and Therapeutics.* Thorofare, NJ: SLACK Incorporated; 1990.)

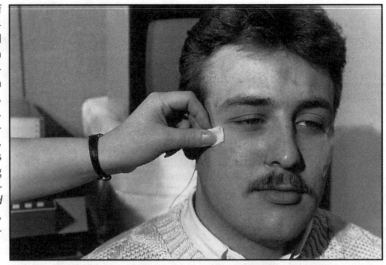

**Figure 6-7.** Next, the skin is carefully abraded with a chemical abrasive and cotton-tip applicator. (Reprinted with permission from Benes SC, McKinney K, Sanders LC, Miller M, Moberg M. *Advanced Ophthalmic Diagnostics and Therapeutics.* Thorofare, NJ: SLACK Incorporated; 1990.)

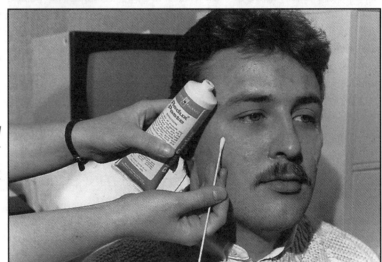

**Figure 6-8.** The cup of the skin electrode is filled with a conductive cream. (Reprinted with permission from Benes SC, McKinney K, Sanders LC, Miller M, Moberg M. *Advanced Ophthalmic Diagnostics and Therapeutics.* Thorofare, NJ: SLACK Incorporated; 1990.)

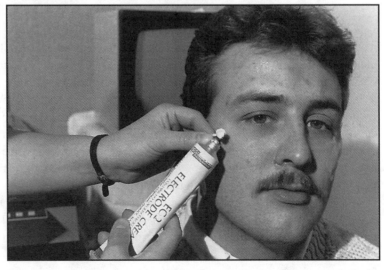

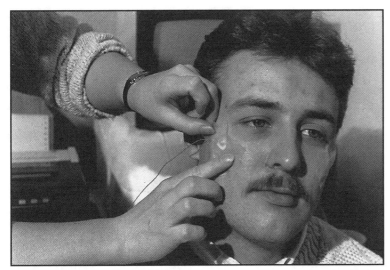

**Figure 6-9.** The skin electrode is firmly attached to the skin with a non-allergenic tape. (Reprinted with permission from Benes SC, McKinney K, Sanders LC, Miller M, Moberg M. *Advanced Ophthalmic Diagnostics and Therapeutics.* Thorofare, NJ: SLACK Incorporated; 1990.)

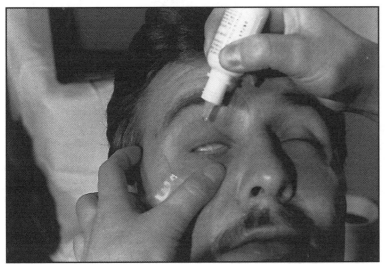

**Figure 6-10.** The eyes are anesthetized. (Reprinted with permission from Benes SC, McKinney K, Sanders LC, Miller M, Moberg M. *Advanced Ophthalmic Diagnostics and Therapeutics.* Thorofare, NJ: SLACK Incorporated; 1990.)

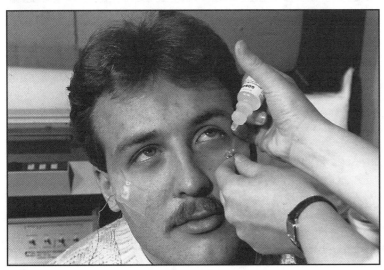

**Figure 6-11.** Methylcellulose is placed inside the corneal contact lens electrode, taking care to exclude air bubbles. (Reprinted with permission from Benes SC, McKinney K, Sanders LC, Miller M, Moberg M. *Advanced Ophthalmic Diagnostics and Therapeutics.* Thorofare, NJ: SLACK Incorporated; 1990.)

**Figure 6-12.** A close-up of two Jet corneal contact lens electrodes in place. They are well centered so the patient can see through them. The wires are left lax and loop outward and then back towards the face where they are secured with tape. (Reprinted with permission from Benes SC, McKinney K, Sanders LC, Miller M, Moberg M. *Advanced Ophthalmic Diagnostics and Therapeutics.* Thorofare, NJ: SLACK Incorporated; 1990.)

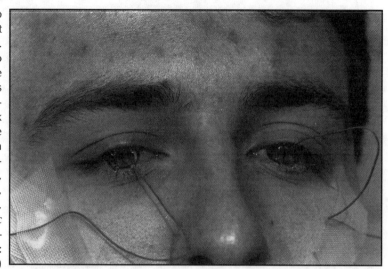

**Figure 6-13.** The patient is now properly prepared for the ERG. The ground electrode is attached behind the ear (not visible in photograph). (Reprinted with permission from Benes SC, McKinney K, Sanders LC, Miller M, Moberg M. *Advanced Ophthalmic Diagnostics and Therapeutics.* Thorofare, NJ: SLACK Incorporated; 1990.)

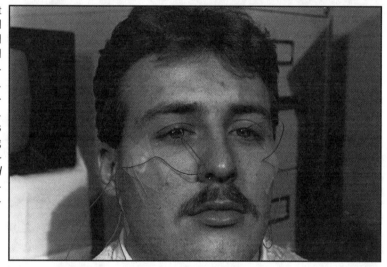

has a speculum attached to it, have the patient look down and slip the upper speculum under the upper lid. Then ask the patient to look up and slip the lower speculum under the lower lid. If the active electrode is a Jet contact lens electrode or one of the other monopolar conductive material electrodes, place a reference electrode above each eye using a similar procedure as that used for the ground electrode. (The patient will then have three skin electrodes on the face—one on the forehead and one above each eye.) The reference electrode can also be placed below and temporal to the eye.

If the patient is going to wear the Jet contact lens electrode, ask him or her to look straight ahead while you pull the lids apart slightly with one hand. With the other hand, put the contact lens directly on the cornea. Again, remind the patient not to squeeze the eye, as the lids may be able to go over the little pegs that are on the outside of this electrode. (They are designed to keep the eye open during testing.) (See Figures 6-6 through 6-13.)

If a gold foil or silver carpet fiber electrode is used, have the patient look up slightly while

## The Scotopic ERG

While in the dark, the patient is stimulated with a very dim flashing light that is presented at intervals of no more than once every 2 seconds. This stimulus is used to elicit a rod response referred to as a scotopic ERG. Four to 16 flashes are presented to obtain the final, averaged scotopic response. Some units use a blue filter to dim the light stimulus, while others use a neutral density filter that is about 2.5 log units less bright than the stimulus used to elicit a cone response. (Cone response will be discussed shortly.) The filters are placed over the same light that is used to elicit a cone response, but the filter cuts out most of the light resulting in a rod-isolated response. Most units have the appropriate filters built into the Ganzfeld bowl. The filters can be changed automatically by changing parameters in the ERG computer program. The typical scotopic response may have either a small a-wave and large b-wave, or only a b-wave (Figure 6-14).

## The Mesopic ERG

A maximal retinal response, referred to as a mesopic ERG, is obtained next. While still in the dark, the patient is stimulated with the light once every 2 seconds, this time without the neutral density or blue filter. Four to 16 flashes are presented to obtain the final, averaged mesopic response. This results in a maximal retinal response elicited by both rods and cones. The rods influence the amplitude of the waveform, while the cones influence the shape of the waveform (Figure 6-15). Other filters (such as red) can be used to stimulate the dark-adapted retina, but these are not necessary for a standard ERG.

## Recording Oscillatory Potentials

While the patient is still dark-adapted, the oscillatory responses should be recorded. These are small waveforms generated by the mid-layers of the retina. The eye is stimulated with the brightest light available without using any filters. The patient is stimulated four times, once every 15 seconds according to International ERG standards. The only thing that really changes is the recording parameters within the computer. Most commercially available programs will come with these parameters already in place. The computer filters out the large amplitude of the retinal response and only records the small wavelets that are seen along the ascending portion of the mesopic ERG b-wave (Figure 6-16). These waveforms are important features of a healthy retina. Their absence can be indicative of early retinal abnormality.

# Recording a Light-Adapted ERG

In order to record a light-adapted ERG, the room lights and the background light in the Ganzfeld bowl must both be turned on. The background luminance of the bowl is designed to suppress the response of rods during light-adapted conditions and should be about 5 to 10 fL (foot lamberts) in strength. Most Ganzfeld bowls will produce this luminance level. Since the patient has been dark-adapted for quite some time, it is important that he or she be light-adapted for at least 5 minutes prior to recording the photopic ERG. If the patient is not adequately light-adapted, a sub-optimal response may be recorded. It is advisable to slowly light-adapt the patient in order to maintain patient comfort, and to then allow the patient to light-adapt for an additional 5 minutes. After adaptation, a photopic ERG can be recorded.

## The Photopic ERG

The photopic ERG is a cone-dominant response. The Ganzfeld bowl is illuminated and a bright light (standard flash without neutral density filters) is used to elicit a cone-dominant

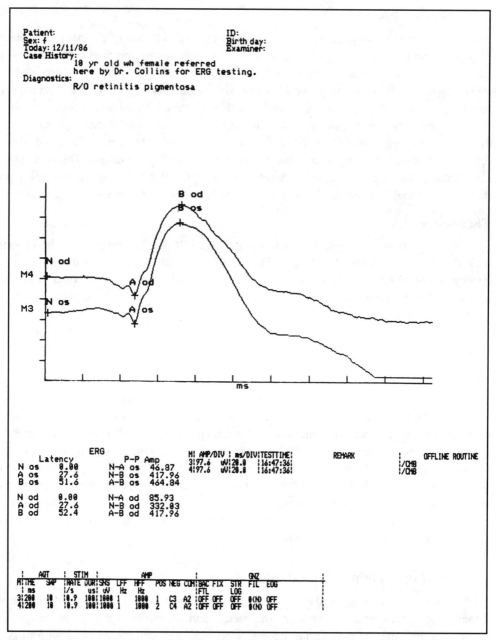

**Figure 6-14.** A typical scotopic ERG. The scotopic ERG is a rod-driven response. The patient has been dark adapted for 30 minutes and is then tested in the dark using a very dim white light. A dim light with a blue filter in front of it can also elicit a similar-looking response. A very small a-wave and large, slow b-wave are typical of scotopic responses. Some scotopic responses have no visible a-wave at all and this is also typical of scotopic ERGs. (Reprinted with permission from Benes SC, McKinney K, Sanders LC, Miller M, Moberg M. *Advanced Ophthalmic Diagnostics and Therapeutics.* Thorofare, NJ: SLACK Incorporated; 1990.)

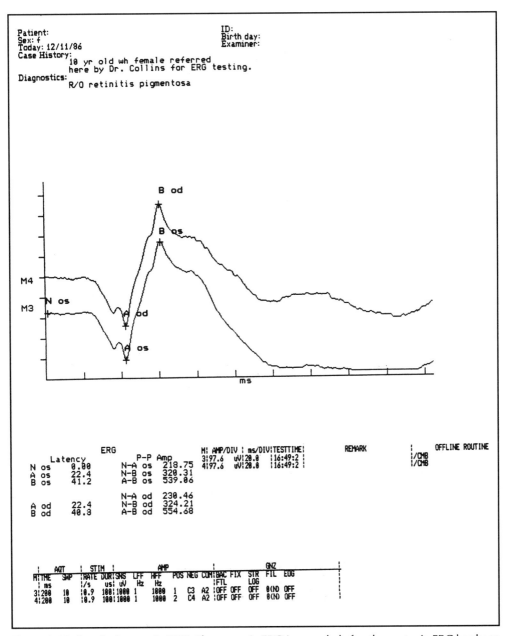

**Figure 6-15.** A typical mesopic ERG. The mesopic ERG is recorded after the scotopic ERG has been recorded. The patient is tested in the dark with a bright light (the same intensity that is used to elicit a cone response). A large a-wave and large, fast b-wave are typical of mesopic responses. The mesopic response looks similar to a photopic ERG that has been "stretched." The mesopic ERG represents both rod and cone function. The rods contribute to the amplitude of the response, whereas the cones contribute to the waveform's general appearance. (Reprinted with permission from Benes SC, McKinney K, Sanders LC, Miller M, Moberg M. *Advanced Ophthalmic Diagnostics and Therapeutics.* Thorofare, NJ: SLACK Incorporated; 1990.)

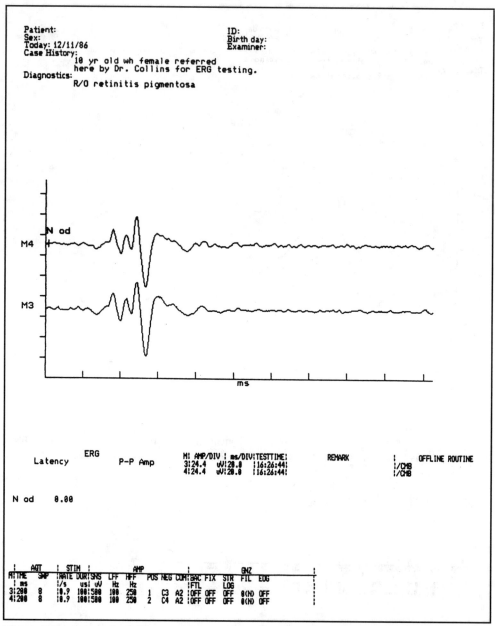

**Figure 6-16.** A typical oscillatory potential. The patient is tested in a dark-adapted state with a bright light. The setting on the machine eliminates the large a- and b-waves, leaving only the small wavelets seen in this illustration. (Reprinted with permission from Benes SC, McKinney K, Sanders LC, Miller M, Moberg M. *Advanced Ophthalmic Diagnostics and Therapeutics.* Thorofare, NJ: SLACK Incorporated; 1990.)

response (Figure 6-17). The response is elicited with either a single flash or with several flashes averaged together. If an averaged cone response is recorded, the rate of stimulation should be about 3 flashes per second.

### The Flicker Fusion ERG

The flicker fusion ERG is a cone-isolated response. The patient is stimulated with the bright light while the background illumination is on. The rate of stimulation is 30 times per second (referred to as 30 hertz [Hz]), and responses are averaged. Only the cones generate this response (between 16 and 32 flashes is optimal) (Figure 6-18).

The rods are not able to fire and re-fire in response to the fast stimulus, while cones can easily fire and re-fire under such conditions. The rate of stimulation can be anywhere from 10 to 95 Hz, but must include a 30 Hz response in order to comply with international standards. The term *flicker fusion* means two things. First, it suggests a point at which the cones do not appreciate the flickering of the light, thus the light appears "on" to them and they are no longer able to fire in response to individual flashes. Also, the person no longer sees the light flickering and now perceives that the light is "on." This is a perceptual fusion of the light, since the light in fact is still flickering. In most normal individuals the flicker fusion level is between 90 and 95 Hz. Young individuals with healthy retinas are usually the ones that produce a flicker response to the 90 Hz stimulus. However, most individuals who are stimulated with a 95 Hz stimulus will produce a non-recordable ERG. In persons with abnormal cone function, their sense of the light being "on" either physiologically or psychophysically may be at a lower frequency than that of a person with normal cone function. Frequently an individual with early cone dysfunction will produce a normal 30 Hz response and a non-recordable 60 Hz response.

### The Red Filter Photopic ERG

A flicker fusion ERG is contraindicated in some individuals. Patients with severe photophobia may not tolerate a flicker fusion ERG. Also, an individual with a seizure disorder (such as epilepsy) may have a seizure if exposed to the rapidly flashing lights. In such instances, a photopic ERG can be obtained by using a red colored filter in front of the white stimulus (Figure 6-19). This results in a cone-isolated ERG. The red filter photopic ERG can be used to isolate cones when other methods are impractical, and will be non-recordable in situations when flicker fusion ERGs would also be non-recordable. The response can be averaged for those with photophobia, or recorded using a single flash for those with epilepsy.

## Concluding the ERG Testing Session

At the end of the procedure, the patient should have the active electrodes removed from his or her eyes. The reference and ground electrodes should also be carefully removed and the excess paste cleaned from the skin with a wet cloth. The patient should be encouraged not to touch or rub the eyes, since they will likely remain numb for several minutes after the end of the examination. The eyes should be washed with an irrigating solution to remove excess methylcellulose. The patient should be warned that the vision will remain blurry for the next hour or so as a result of the procedure and that the blurriness is a normal side effect. The patient should be told that the eyes may feel a little uncomfortable for the next several hours but should not be painful. If the eyes do feel painful he or she should either return to the clinic or seek attention from the referring ophthalmologist. Pain may indicate a corneal abrasion, an extremely rare side effect of ERG testing that may occur if the patient fails to heed your warning about not rubbing the eyes.

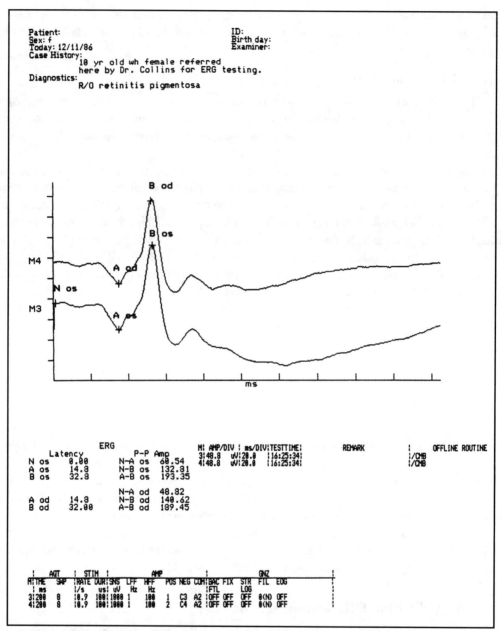

**Figure 6-17.** A typical photopic ERG. The photopic ERG is recorded after the oscillatory potential. The patient is light-adapted for at least five minutes prior to photopic ERG testing. Care must be taken to insure that the patient is light-adapted for at least five minutes since less time will result in an ERG that is abnormally low in amplitude. The amplitude reduction is a result of insufficient light adaptation and not disease. The photopic ERG is comprised of a fast a-wave followed by a fast, but low amplitude, b-wave. (Reprinted with permission from Benes SC, McKinney K, Sanders LC, Miller M, Moberg M. *Advanced Ophthalmic Diagnostics and Therapeutics.* Thorofare, NJ: SLACK Incorporated; 1990.)

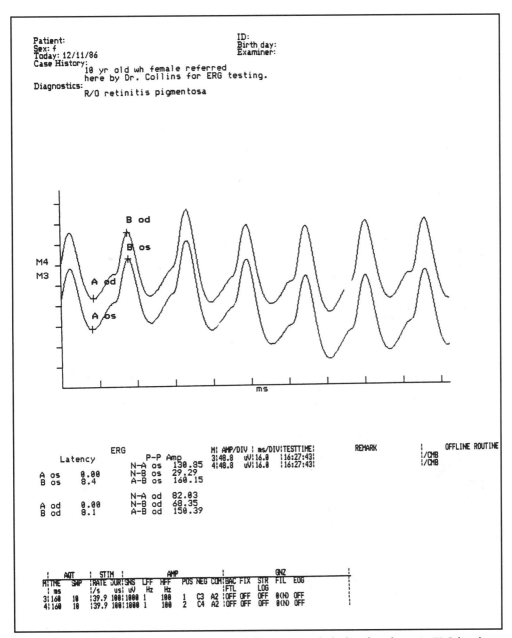

**Figure 6-18.** A typical flicker ERG. The flicker ERG is recorded after the photopic ERG has been recorded. The patient remains in a light-adapted state and is stimulated with a bright light that is presented at a 30Hz rate (30 times per second). This results in a response that is driven solely by cones, as the rods cannot respond to the quick flashing light. The flicker ERG looks like numerous photopic ERGs lined up next to each other. The b-wave amplitude is the most important measurement to take from this particular waveform. (Reprinted with permission from Benes SC, McKinney K, Sanders LC, Miller M, Moberg M. *Advanced Ophthalmic Diagnostics and Therapeutics.* Thorofare, NJ: SLACK Incorporated; 1990.)

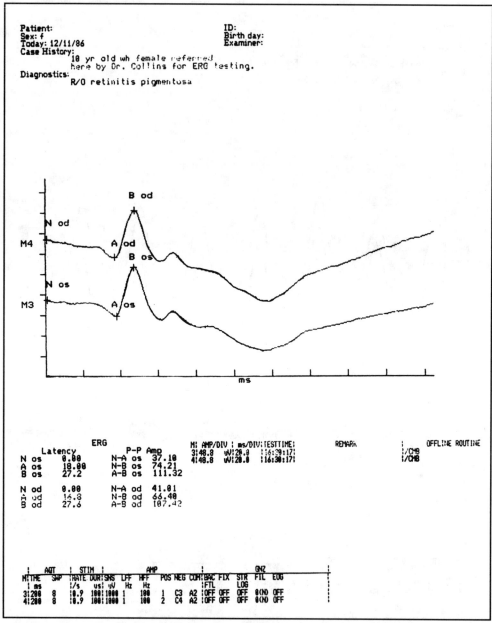

**Figure 6-19.** A typical red filter photopic ERG. The red filter photopic ERG represents only cone activity as does the flicker ERG. This response can be recorded when a flicker ERG is contraindicated (as in the case of patients with epilepsy) or can be used to verify amplitude reduction in flicker ERGs. The red filter photopic ERG has a lower amplitude and slight simplification in waveform as compared with a standard photopic ERG, but still has the typical appearance of both the a- and b-waves. (Reprinted with permission from Benes SC, McKinney K, Sanders LC, Miller M, Moberg M. *Advanced Ophthalmic Diagnostics and Therapeutics.* Thorofare, NJ: SLACK Incorporated; 1990.)

# Results of ERG Testing

## The ERG Waveform

There are several components of the ERG waveform. The first component is a cornea-negative waveform referred to as an "a-wave." The photoreceptor cell layer within the retina generates this response. The second component is a cornea-positive response that is referred to as a "b-wave." This response is generated by the mid-retinal layers, primarily the Müller and bipolar cells.

These two waveforms are superimposed on one another to produce an ERG. The a and b-waves are measured for amplitude and peak delay. The amplitude of the a-wave is measured from the baseline at the stimulus artifact to the trough of the a-wave as depicted in Figure 6-20. The amplitude of the b-wave is measured from the trough of the a-wave to the peak of the b-wave (see Figure 6-20).

The peak delay, also known as implicit time (but frequently interchanged with the term latency), is measured from onset of the stimulus to the peak of the b-wave. The true latency of the waveform is measured from the stimulus to the beginning of either the a- or b-waves. The beginning of the b-wave occurs at the trough of the a-wave, but this is difficult to measure, so many individuals refer to the distance from the stimulus onset to the peak of the b-wave as b-wave latency. (This is not an accurate measurement of latency, but is a term frequently used, and easiest to understand. Peak delay and latency will be used interchangeably throughout this text.) These measurements are used to determine if the retinal response is within or outside the normal range.

There are several other components of the ERG waveform, including a "c-wave" that is generated by the RPE, but this is a difficult waveform to record in a clinical setting. The c-wave of the ERG occurs at just about the same time as when a patient blinks in response to the flash of light. Thus, what generally is recorded is a blink response and not a c-wave. So unless the patient is sedated and will not respond to the flashing light by blinking, it is not practical to try to record this waveform. Electro-oculography (see Chapter 7) is a much easier means by which to assess RPE function. Within a clinical setting, the a- and b-waves are the most useful for assessing retinal activity.

The ERG waveform will look different depending on the type of photoreceptor that is stimulated during testing. The retinal response can be either from cones (photopic, flicker fusion, or red filter), rods (scotopic), or cones and rods (mesopic). The photopic ERG has a fast a and b-wave, and is a fairly small response. The amplitude of the b-wave is about 100 μv (microvolts) and the peak delay of the b-wave is about 22 msecs (milliseconds). The scotopic ERG has almost no discernible a-wave, but has a slow b-wave that has a peak delay of about 60 msecs and an amplitude of about 200 μv. The mesopic ERG looks like an elongated photopic response. The shape of the waveform is driven by the cones, whereas the amplitude of the wave is driven by the rods. The peak delay of the b-wave is about 35 msecs, and the amplitude from the trough of the a-wave to the peak of the b-wave is about 350 μv. Figures 6-14 to 6-19, already referred to in the text, illustrate the various ERGs.

## The Abnormal ERG

There are several types of abnormalities that can be observed in a standard ERG. They include a reduction in ERG amplitude, a slowing of the waveform (shift in latency and peak delay), and

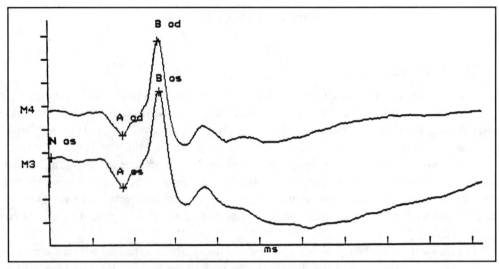

**Figure 6-20.** This photopic ERG is marked for measuring the amplitude and latency of the waves. The vertical axis represents microvolts and the horizontal axis represents milliseconds. The divisions (tick marks) along each axis are pre-determined by the computer. The computer is able to automatically measure the amplitude and latency of both the a- and b-waves. This is done by moving the cursor to the trough of the a-wave and to the peak of the b-wave (where the small crosses are located on the tracing). The latency of the response is measured by the computer in milliseconds from the time the flash occurred until the trough of the a-wave or the peak of the b-wave is present. A delay in waveform latency can indicate generalized retinal disease (such as retinitis pigmentosa). The amplitude of the a-wave is measured from the baseline (straight line noted prior to the downward deflection of the a-wave) to the trough of the a-wave. The amplitude of the b-wave is measured in microvolts from the trough of the a-wave to the peak of the b-wave. A reduced amplitude ERG would be consistent with some type of retinal pathology such as retinal detachment. Similar calculations for the scotopic and mesopic waveforms can be made by the computer and the calculations are based on the measurement techniques just described. (The measurement of the scotopic ERG does not include an a-wave measurement, as there is rarely an a-wave visible in the tracing.) (Reprinted with permission from Benes SC, McKinney K, Sanders LC, Miller M, Moberg M. *Advanced Ophthalmic Diagnostics and Therapeutics.* Thorofare, NJ: SLACK Incorporated; 1990.)

a reduction in b-wave amplitude without evidence of a-wave involvement (shift to negativity). The reduction in ERG amplitude (both a- and b-waves) suggests that some portion of the retina is non-functioning, but that the remaining retina is functioning normally. This is frequently seen in such disorders as retinal detachment. A slowing of the waveform suggests that the photoreceptor cells are firing abnormally slowly. This is seen in degenerative disorders of the retina such as retinitis pigmentosa or choroideremia. There can be a reduction in b-wave amplitude with normal a-wave values, as seen in mid-retinal layer abnormalities (involving Müller and/or bipolar cells) such as retinoschisis.

Additional findings include supernormal amplitudes, where the amplitude is several standard deviations greater than the mean ERG amplitude. This can be seen in such disorders as ocular albinism or very early retinal degeneration. A normal ERG can be recorded in individuals with focal retinal pathology, as in macular degeneration. A non-recordable ERG can result when less than 10% of the total retinal area is capable of generating an ERG, as in end-stage retinitis pigmentosa.

Finally, cone-only or rod-only abnormalities might be observed. In the cone-only abnormality, the individual will often complain of loss of visual acuity, photophobia, and poor color vision. In widespread cone disease the photopic, flicker fusion, and red filter photopic ERGs will all be abnormal or non-recordable but the scotopic ERG will be normal. This can be seen in patients with cone dystrophy. In a rod-only abnormality, the individual will often complain of night blindness and visual field constriction. In widespread rod disease the scotopic ERG will be abnormal or non-recordable, and the mesopic ERG will be reduced in amplitude, but the photopic ERG may be within the normal range. This can be seen in patients with a rod dystrophy or congenital stationary night blindness.

# The Clinical Usefulness of the ERG

It may be quite apparent from the discussion of ERG waveform abnormalities that the test can be clinically useful in the evaluation of retinal disorders. Certainly, some retinal abnormalities can be determined based on funduscopic presentation and chief complaints alone. However, the ERG can be an excellent adjunct to these clinical presentations.

The ERG can be used to differentiate between widespread and localized retinal disease, to determine if both the rods and cones or only the rods or cones are involved, to help establish whether the abnormality is progressive or stationary, and for establishing visual prognosis in individuals with retinal degenerative disorders. Finally, the ERG can be useful in the evaluation of unexplained vision loss, especially in infants and young children.

Several case histories will be presented to illustrate the three basic waveform abnormalities of loss of amplitude, slowing, and shift to negativity. This will be followed by several case studies that will illustrate the usefulness of the ERG in determining which photoreceptor cells are involved, whether the disorder is localized or generalized, whether the abnormality is stationary or progressive, and the possible visual prognosis of several individuals with these various disorders. Three case studies of unexplained vision loss in infants and young children will conclude this chapter.

# Case Histories—Basic Waveform Abnormalities

## 6-1. Retinal Detachment

The patient was a 70-year-old male with a history of possible rhegmatogenous retinal detachment, OS. There was not a good view of the posterior pole due to the presence of a dense cataract. An ultrasound suggested both a posterior vitreous detachment and a retinal detachment. He was sent for ERG testing to rule out a retinal detachment.

An ERG was recorded under standard conditions (Figure 6-21). The left eye (bottom tracing) shows both a normal photopic and scotopic response. The response from the right eye is abnormal—both the photopic and scotopic responses are reduced in amplitude by about 50% (upper tracing). However, the peak delay of the b-wave under both conditions of testing is the same for both eyes. This suggests that part of the right retina is non-functioning, but that the remaining retina is functioning normally (there is no evidence of slowing of the waveform). The 50% loss of amplitude from the right eye as compared to the left eye suggests that about 50% of the right retina is non-functioning. This would be consistent with a 50% retinal detachment. This type of

**Figure 6-21.** ERG from patient with a retinal detachment of the left eye. Note the reduction in amplitude of the affected eye as compared to the normal eye. The amplitude is reduced by approximately 50%, suggesting a 50% retinal detachment. The peak of both the photopic and scotopic b-waves are identical between the two eyes, suggesting that the remaining retina is functioning normally, as would be the case in retinal detachments. (Illustration courtesy of Thomas E. Ogden, MD, PhD.)

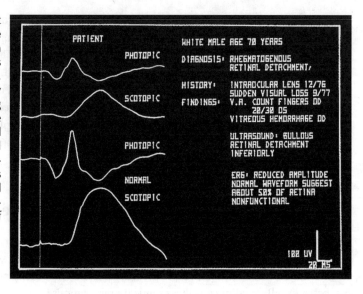

waveform abnormality would not be associated with a posterior vitreous detachment (as was suggested by the ultrasound), as the ERG is not affected by vitreous detachments. Therefore, the ERG was necessary to make the diagnosis of retinal detachment in this patient.

## 6-2. Early Retinitis Pigmentosa

The patient was a 68-year-old male, who had few visual complaints. He went in for a routine eye examination and was found to have funduscopic changes similar to those seen in individuals with retinitis pigmentosa. The patient reported that he had recently noted some mild problems with night vision, but did not really think of them as serious and felt that they were a normal part of aging. He was sent for ERG testing.

An ERG was recorded under standard conditions. The ERG under both photopic and scotopic conditions of testing showed normal b-wave amplitudes, but revealed abnormal b-wave latency. Figure 6-22 shows that the b-waves were delayed by about 10 msecs under both photopic and scotopic conditions, suggesting the presence of an early retinal degeneration and a probable diagnosis of early retinitis pigmentosa. (This was confirmed by dark adaptometry testing, which revealed a final rod threshold that was 1.5 log units above normal. See the section on dark adaptometry in Chapter 2 for details of this test.)

These findings were present prior to any real visual complaints from the patient. Due to his age, it is likely that the abnormality is very slowly progressing and that he will never have any functional deficits as a result of retinitis pigmentosa. If he does have a functional deficit, it will be noted only when he is very old. Thus, his ocular prognosis is quite good.

## 6-3. Retinoschisis Versus Retinal Detachment

The patient is a 33-year-old male with a longstanding history of poor vision; he has a sibling with similar problems. Funduscopic examination revealed possible bilateral retinal detachments. He was sent for ERG testing.

An ERG was recorded under standard conditions. The responses under photopic and mesopic conditions were abnormal and revealed a loss of b-wave amplitudes and normal a-wave ampli-

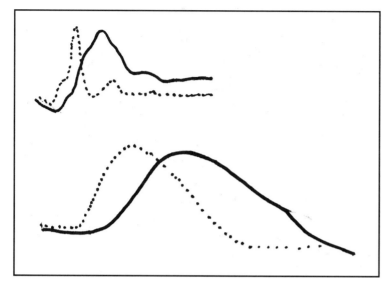

**Figure 6-22.** ERG from patient with early retinitis pigmentosa. The first change in the ERG is a prolongation of latency, referred to as *slowing*, as a result of abnormal firing of the photoreceptor cells. Later there will also be a reduction in amplitude, suggesting a dying off of photoreceptor cells. The dotted line is a normal ERG (for reference) and the solid line is the patient's abnormal ERG showing slowing.

tudes without evidence of slowing (Figure 6-23). The scotopic ERG showed a severe loss of b-wave amplitudes from both eyes. These findings would be consistent with a diagnosis of bilateral retinoschisis, where the photoreceptor cells and mid-retinal layers detach from one another, thus leaving a normal photoreceptor cell response (a-wave) and an abnormal Müller and bipolar cell response (b-wave). (Both a- and b-waves would have been reduced if retinal detachments had been present.)

# Case Histories—Disorders Suggesting Cone Photoreceptor Cell Abnormality

## 6-4. Cone Dystrophy Versus Stargardt's Disease

The patient was a 17-year-old female with a 6-month history of decreased vision OU, poor color perception, and mild photophobia. She presented with macular changes in both eyes. She was sent for ERG testing to evaluate the retinal function of both eyes. Provisional diagnosis was cone dystrophy versus Stargardt's disease. (Stargardt's disease is a juvenile-onset macular degeneration that is localized to the photoreceptors of the macula, whereas cone dystrophy affects all of the cones throughout the retina.)

An ERG was recorded under standard conditions. The tracings in Figure 6-24 revealed normal photopic and scotopic responses in both eyes. The results suggest a localized abnormality confined to the macular area (with less than 1% retinal involvement). Her overall visual prognosis is quite good, as the retinal abnormality should not progress beyond the macular area.

## 6-5. Cone Dystrophy Versus Stargardt's Disease

The patient was a 16-year-old male with a 6-month history of decreased vision OU, poor color perception, and mild photophobia. He presented with macular changes in both eyes. He was

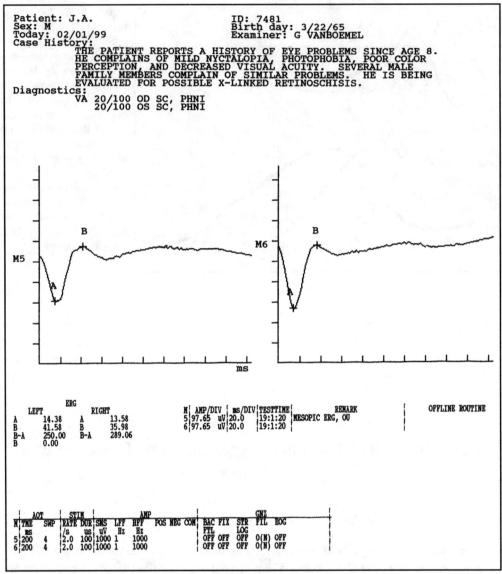

```
Patient: J.A.                    ID: 7481
Sex: M                           Birth day: 3/22/65
Today: 02/01/99                  Examiner: G VANBOEMEL
Case History:
          THE PATIENT REPORTS A HISTORY OF EYE PROBLEMS SINCE AGE 8.
          HE COMPLAINS OF MILD NYCTALOPIA, PHOTOPHOBIA, POOR COLOR
          PERCEPTION, AND DECREASED VISUAL ACUITY.  SEVERAL MALE
          FAMILY MEMBERS COMPLAIN OF SIMILAR PROBLEMS.  HE IS BEING
          EVALUATED FOR POSSIBLE X-LINKED RETINOSCHISIS.
Diagnostics:
          VA  20/100 OD SC, PHNI
              20/100 OS SC, PHNI
```

```
            ERG
       LEFT         RIGHT       N  AMP/DIV   ms/DIV TESTTIME            REMARK              OFFLINE ROUTINE
A      14.38    A    13.58      5  97.65 uV  20.0   19:1:20  MESOPIC ERG, OU
B      41.58    B    35.98      6  97.65 uV  20.0   19:1:20
B-A   250.00    B-A 289.06
B       0.00
```

```
      AOT       STIM              AMP                        GNZ
N  TME   SWP  RATE DUR SNS LFF HFF  POS NEG CON  BAC FIX  STR FIL  EOG
   ms         /s   us  uV  Hz  Hz                FTL      LOG
5  200    4   2.0  100 1000 1  1000         OFF OFF  OFF O(N) OFF
6  200    4   2.0  100 1000 1  1000         OFF OFF  OFF O(N) OFF
```

**Figure 6-23.** Mesopic ERG from a patient with retinoschisis. The a-wave is normal, whereas the b-wave is very abnormal in amplitude, suggesting that the Müller and bi-polar cells are not firing but the photoreceptor cells are functioning normally. This is referred to as a *negative* waveform.

sent for ERG testing to evaluate retinal function. Provisional diagnosis was cone dystrophy versus Stargardt's disease.

An ERG was recorded under standard conditions. The tracings in Figure 6-25 revealed normal scotopic response. The photopic ERG was abnormal. (Note the reduction in amplitude and slowing of the top waveform. A normal photopic ERG (middle tracing) is included for reference.) The results suggest a widespread cone abnormality consistent with a diagnosis of cone dystrophy in which all of the cone photoreceptors are affected. His visual prognosis is poor, since all of his cones are affected. He will ultimately have extremely poor daytime vision and

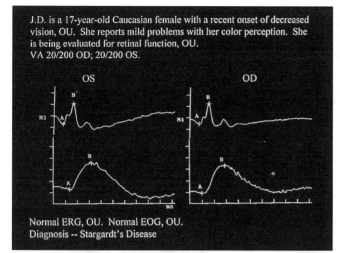

J.D. is a 17-year-old Caucasian female with a recent onset of decreased vision, OU. She reports mild problems with her color perception. She is being evaluated for retinal function, OU.
VA 20/200 OD; 20/200 OS.

OS          OD

Normal ERG, OU. Normal EOG, OU.
Diagnosis -- Stargardt's Disease

**Figure 6-24.** A normal ERG from a patient diagnosed with Stargardt's juvenile-onset macular degeneration. The normal response suggests that the abnormality is localized to the macular area only and does not involve the entire retina.

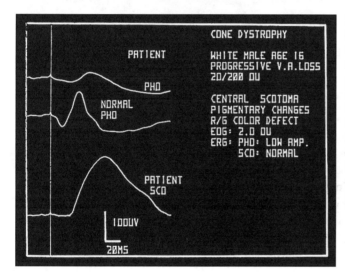

CONE DYSTROPHY

PATIENT

PHO

NORMAL
PHO

PATIENT
SCO

1 00UV

20MS

WHITE MALE AGE 16
PROGRESSIVE V.A.LOSS
20/200 OU

CENTRAL SCOTOMA
PIGMENTARY CHANGES
R/G COLOR DEFECT
EOG: 2.0 OU
ERG: PHO: LOW AMP.
SCO: NORMAL

**Figure 6-25.** An abnormal photopic ERG from a patient with a diagnosis of cone dystrophy. The symptoms are similar to that of a person with Stargardt's disease; however the ERG findings suggest that all of the cone cells are involved, not just the ones in the macular area. The normal photopic ERG is present as a comparison against which the abnormal photopic ERG (top one) can be judged. (Illustration courtesy of Thomas E. Ogden, MD, PhD.)

will eventually lose all of his color perception, leaving him with achromatic (black and white only) vision.

## 6-6. Congenital Achromatopsia Versus Cone Dystrophy

The patient was a 29-year-old female with a history of poor vision for as long as she could remember. Her visual acuity was 20/200 in each eye. She complained of mild photophobia and a complete absence of color perception (she saw only in black and white), and she presented with fine horizontal nystagmus. She reported that her vision has been stable all of her life. She was sent for ERG testing to evaluate the retinal function of both eyes.

An ERG was recorded under standard conditions. The tracings in Figure 6-26 revealed normal scotopic responses in both eyes. The photopic ERGs were non-recordable in both eyes. The results suggest widespread cone abnormality consistent with some type of cone dystrophy. The fact that she has had these symptoms all of her life suggests that they are congenital. Also, she

**Figure 6-26.** A non-recordable photopic ERG from a patient with achromatopsia (rod monochromatism). The photopic ERG is nonrecordable as the patient is born with no cones. These individuals have severely reduced vision from birth, a virtual absence of color perception, difficulty seeing in the daytime, and non-recordable photopic ERG.

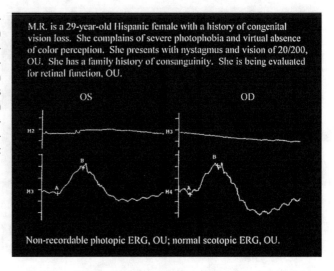

M.R. is a 29-year-old Hispanic female with a history of congenital vision loss. She complains of severe photophobia and virtual absence of color perception. She presents with nystagmus and vision of 20/200, OU. She has a family history of consanguinity. She is being evaluated for retinal function, OU.

Non-recordable photopic ERG, OU; normal scotopic ERG, OU.

did not report any progression of abnormality. This suggests a diagnosis of congenital achromatopsia, in which the individual is born without cone photoreceptor cells.

## 6-7. Cone/Rod Dystrophy

The patient was an 11-year-old male with a history of decreased vision, and mild photophobia for the past five years. He was sent for ERG testing to evaluate retinal function of both eyes.

An ERG was recorded under standard conditions. The tracings in Figure 6-27 revealed a severely abnormal photopic ERG in both eyes. The scotopic responses were also abnormal, consisting of a loss of b-wave amplitude, slowing, and a shift to negativity. The results suggest a widespread retinal abnormality involving both cones and rods, but cones more than rods. The findings would be consistent with a diagnosis of cone/rod dystrophy. His visual prognosis is very poor and he will ultimately have extremely poor daytime and nighttime vision, and may eventually become totally blind as a result of the disorder.

# Case Histories—Disorders Suggesting Rod Photoreceptor Cell Abnormality

## 6-8. Congenital Stationary Night Blindness

The patient was a 25-year-old male who reported a history of nyctalopia for as long as he could remember. He reported visual field constriction that occurred only in the dark. Funduscopic findings were essentially normal in both eyes. He was sent for ERG testing to evaluate retinal function of both eyes.

An ERG was recorded under standard conditions. The tracings in Figure 6-28 revealed a normal photopic ERG. His scotopic ERG was severely abnormal (middle tracing). The results suggest a widespread retinal abnormality involving only the rods. The history and findings would be consistent with a diagnosis of congenital stationary night blindness, where the individual is born

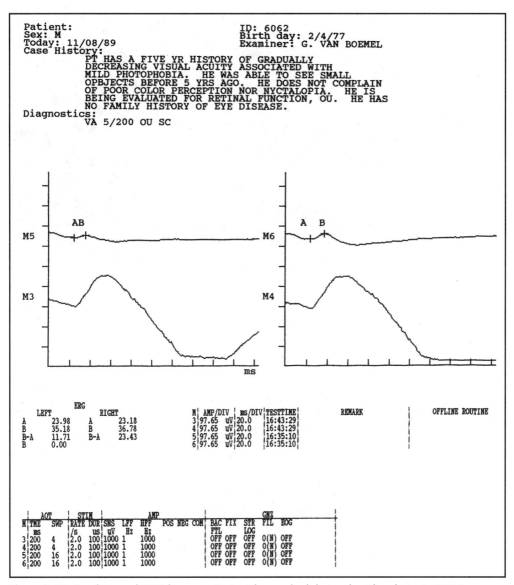

```
Patient:                        ID: 6062
Sex: M                          Birth day: 2/4/77
Today: 11/08/89                 Examiner: G. VAN BOEMEL
Case History:
          PT HAS A FIVE YR HISTORY OF GRADUALLY
          DECREASING VISUAL ACUITY ASSOCIATED WITH
          MILD PHOTOPHOBIA.  HE WAS ABLE TO SEE SMALL
          OPBJECTS BEFORE 5 YRS AGO.  HE DOES NOT COMPLAIN
          OF POOR COLOR PERCEPTION NOR NYCTALOPIA.  HE IS
          BEING EVALUATED FOR RETINAL FUNCTION, OU.  HE HAS
          NO FAMILY HISTORY OF EYE DISEASE.
Diagnostics:
          VA 5/200 OU SC
```

|  | ERG | | | N | AMP/DIV | | ms/DIV | TESTTIME | | REMARK | | OFFLINE ROUTINE |
|---|---|---|---|---|---|---|---|---|---|---|---|---|
| LEFT | | RIGHT | | | | | | | | | | |
| A | 23.98 | A | 23.18 | 3 | 97.65 | uV | 20.0 | 16:43:29 | | | | |
| B | 35.18 | B | 36.78 | 4 | 97.65 | uV | 20.0 | 16:43:29 | | | | |
| B-A | 11.71 | B-A | 23.43 | 5 | 97.65 | uV | 20.0 | 16:35:10 | | | | |
| B | 0.00 | | | 6 | 97.65 | uV | 20.0 | 16:35:10 | | | | |

| N | AOT | | STIM | | AMP | | | | | | GNZ | | | |
|---|---|---|---|---|---|---|---|---|---|---|---|---|---|---|
| | TIME | SWP | RATE | DUR | SNS | LFF | HPF | POS NEG CON | BAC FIX | STR | FIL | EOG | | |
| | ms | | /s | us | uV | Hz | Hz | | FTL | LOG | | | | |
| 3 | 200 | 4 | 2.0 | 100 | 1000 | 1 | 1000 | | OFF OFF | OFF | O(N) | OFF | | |
| 4 | 200 | 4 | 2.0 | 100 | 1000 | 1 | 1000 | | OFF OFF | OFF | O(N) | OFF | | |
| 5 | 200 | 16 | 2.0 | 100 | 1000 | 1 | 1000 | | OFF OFF | OFF | O(N) | OFF | | |
| 6 | 200 | 16 | 2.0 | 100 | 1000 | 1 | 1000 | | OFF OFF | OFF | O(N) | OFF | | |

**Figure 6-27.** An abnormal ERG from a patient with cone/rod dystrophy. The photopic ERG is severely abnormal and the scotopic ERG is mild to moderately abnormal. This disease would be classified as a cone/rod dystrophy as there is greater involvement of the cones, than the rods.

**Figure 6-28.** An ERG from a patient with congenital stationary night blindness. His scotopic ERG (middle tracing) is severely abnormal (and possibly represents cone function). The patient has severe night blindness that was present from birth. The normal scotopic ERG (bottom tracing) is present as a comparison. (Illustration courtesy of Thomas E. Ogden, MD, PhD.)

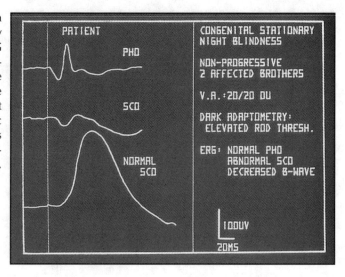

without rod photoreceptor cells. His visual prognosis is better than that of an individual with either cone/rod dystrophy or retinitis pigmentosa, as he will maintain his normal cone function, good visual acuity, and normal color perception the rest of his life (unless he develops other ocular disorders such as glaucoma).

## 6-9. Retinitis Pigmentosa

The patient was a 17-year-old male with a history of nyctalopia and visual field loss for as long as he could remember. He reported that these symptoms had worsened recently, and that his visual acuity and color perception had worsened as well. His visual acuity was about 20/60 OU and his visual fields were about 7 degrees OU. He was being evaluated for retinal function of both eyes.

An ERG was recorded under standard conditions. The tracings in Figure 6-29 revealed a nonrecordable ERG under all conditions of testing. The results suggest a widespread retinal abnormality involving both rods and cones. The findings would be consistent with end-stage retinitis pigmentosa. Because of his age, vision, visual fields, and ERG findings, his prognosis is very poor. Unlike the older patient with only mild retinal changes (see Figure 6-22), this individual will probably be blind before age forty.

## Case Histories—The ERG in Unexplained Vision Loss

### 6-10. Unexplained Vision Loss in an Infant

The patient was a 6-month-old female who had a history of nystagmus and virtually absent visual behavior; otherwise her eye findings were unremarkable. The infant was being evaluated for possible Leber's Congenital Amaurosis (a congenital defect of the retina, resulting in severe reduction in vision or total blindness).

An ERG was recorded under standard conditions with the use of a Burian-Allen contact lens electrode. The tracings in Figure 6-30 revealed an essentially normal ERG under all conditions

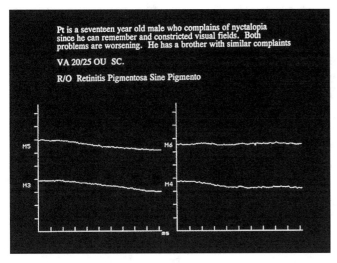

Pt is a seventeen year old male who complains of nyctalopia since he can remember and constricted visual fields. Both problems are worsening. He has a brother with similar complaints

VA 20/25 OU SC.

R/O Retinitis Pigmentosa Sine Pigmento

**Figure 6-29.** A non-recordable ERG from a 17-year-old patient with a history of retinitis pigmentosa. The findings suggest that as little as 10% of his retina is still functioning, as no clear-cut response could be recorded. The visual prognosis for this patient is grim and suggests that he may be totally blind before the age of 30.

of testing. The results do not suggest a widespread retinal abnormality involving either cones or rods. The infant also underwent flash VER testing that was within the normal range. (See Chapter 8 for her VER findings, illustrated in Figure 8-23) The findings are not consistent with a diagnosis of Leber's Congenital Amaurosis in which the infant is born with a non-functional retina. Her visual prognosis is quite good, and it is likely that she has delayed visual maturation OU. Children with normal electrodiagnostic findings and poor visual behavior are considered to be visually delayed, and many will develop normal vision at a later than average time. (Note: Mild ERG changes in a non-sedated, crying infant are not considered clinically significant, as the changes are likely due to movement artifact and not pathology.)

## 6-11. Unexplained Vision Loss in an Infant

The patient was a 9-month-old male, who had a history of nystagmus and virtually absent visual behavior. His parents were concerned because he appeared to "look" at them only when he was able to hear them. The infant was being evaluated for possible Leber's Congenital Amaurosis.

An ERG was recorded under standard conditions. The tracings in Figure 6-31 revealed a non-recordable ERG under all conditions of testing. The results suggest a widespread retinal abnormality involving both rods and cones. The findings would be consistent with a diagnosis of Leber's Congenital Amaurosis. His visual prognosis is extremely poor, and it is likely that he will not have visual acuity that is significantly better than light perception OU. The vision loss is stable in these children, and should not worsen over time.

## 6-12. Unexplained Vision Loss in a Young Child with Previously Normal Vision

The patient was a 3-year-old female who had a history of significant vision loss and nyctalopia over the past 3 months. The mother reported that her daughter's vision had seemed normal when she was 2 years old, but had deteriorated recently. The child was being evaluated for possible retinal abnormality.

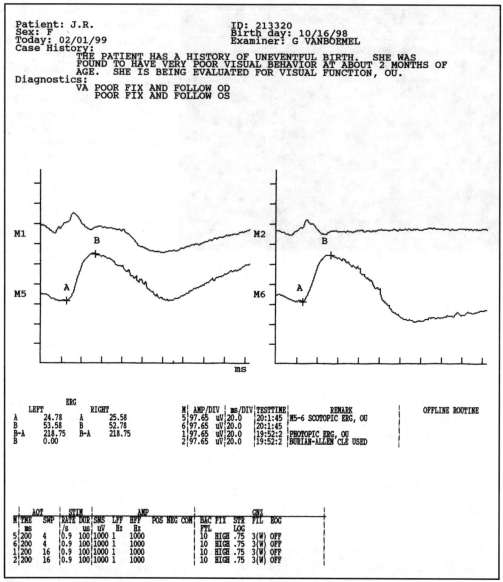

**Figure 6-30.** A normal ERG from a six-month-old child who presented with virtually absent visual behavior. A normal VER was also recorded from this child (see Figure 8-23). The results would be consistent with delayed visual maturation and the child should eventually develop visual behavior. This child was tested while awake, using Burian-Allen corneal contact lens electrodes. Under these conditions, mild changes in amplitude are not considered clinically significant as the changes are probably due to movement artifact (blinking and crying) and not due to ocular pathology. Non-recordable (Figure 6-31) or severely abnormal (Figure 6-32) ERGs would be considered clinically significant, however.

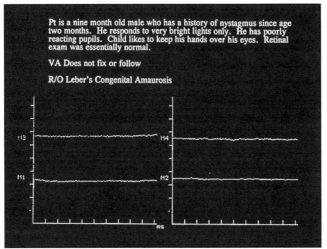

Pt is a nine month old male who has a history of nystagmus since age two months. He responds to very bright lights only. He has poorly reacting pupils. Child likes to keep his hands over his eyes. Retinal exam was essentially normal.

VA Does not fix or follow

R/O Leber's Congenital Amaurosis

**Figure 6-31.** A non-recordable ERG from an infant with Leber's congenital amaurosis. Like the child with delayed visual maturation, this child has virtually no visual behavior. But the absence of visual behavior, in this case, is based on profound retinal pathology. This child's visual behavior will not improve significantly.

An ERG was recorded under standard conditions. The tracings in Figure 6-32 revealed a recordable, but severely abnormal ERG under all conditions of testing. The abnormality consisted of a loss of b-wave amplitude, slowing of the waveform, and shift to negativity (more loss of b-wave amplitude than a-wave amplitude). The results suggest a widespread retinal abnormality involving both rods and cones. The findings would be consistent with retinitis pigmentosa, in which there is notable degeneration of the retina after birth. (Some researchers believe that retinitis pigmentosa in very young children is actually a variant of Leber's Congenital Amaurosis.) Her visual prognosis is extremely poor, and it is likely that she will regress to having no light perception vision by the time she is about 10 years old.

# Reference

1. Marmor MF, Arden GB, Nilsson SEG, and Zrenner E. Standard for clinical electroretinography. *Ach Ophthalmol* 1989;107:816-819.

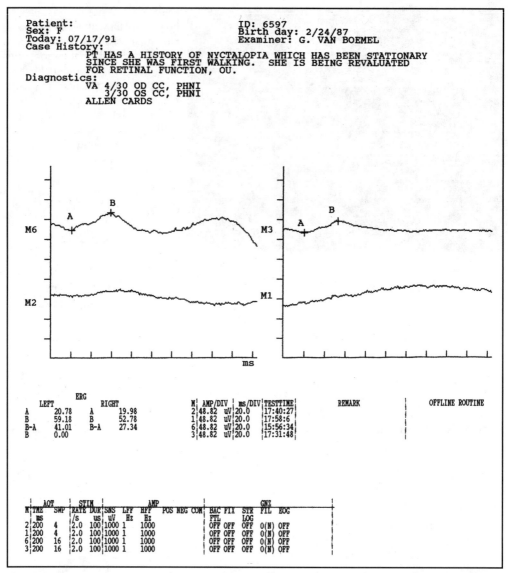

**Figure 6-32.** An ERG from a 3-year-old girl whose mother noted that she had developed night blindness about six months earlier. The ERG on the left is severely abnormal, but recordable. A second ERG recorded one year later (recording on the right) shows additional reduction in photopic ERG amplitude. The second scotopic response is virtually non-recordable. The findings are consistent with a diagnosis such as retinitis pigmentosa.

# Chapter 7

# Electro-Oculography

- The electro-oculogram (EOG) is an indirect test to determine how well the retinal pigment epithelium (RPE) is functioning.

- Unlike the ERG, the EOG is a qualitative test of RPE function.

- The EOG requires good visual acuity and reasonable cooperation on the part of the patient.

- The EOG is an excellent test to use on individuals with suspected retinal abnormalities.

# Introduction to the Electro-Oculogram

The electro-oculogram (EOG) is the easiest of the ocular electrophysiology tests to perform and the most difficult to explain. The EOG is a test that indirectly measures the standing electrical potential that exists between the back and the front of the eye. This standing potential, referred to as the corneo-fundal potential, produces a 6 to 10 microvolt difference between the cornea and the posterior pole. The direction of the current flow is similar to that of the ERG, thus making the cornea more positive relative to the back of the eye.

This voltage difference is particularly noticeable when the eye is in a light-adapted state. In fact, light adaptation actually results in a significant increase (a doubling of the potential in a light-adapted state as compared to an eye in a dark-adapted state) in the corneo-fundal potential in a normal eye. Originally, the standing potential measured by means of the EOG was thought to be produced by the lens, cornea, ciliary body, and RPE. Through later experimentation it was found that the actual origin of the standing potential was from the RPE and the photoreceptors. Therefore the EOG can produce reliable information that can be helpful in the diagnosis of retinal degenerative disorders.

A simple way to explain the current flow in the eye is to think of the eye as a battery. As mentioned before, there is a measurable voltage difference between the back and front of the eye. In addition, the eye "runs down" in the dark and "recharges" in the light. In order for this battery-like effect to occur, a barrier must be present between the two poles (the back and the front of the eye). That barrier happens to be the RPE. The cells of the RPE have very tight junctions resulting in a blood-retina barrier. Since it is impossible to put a volt meter on the back and front of the patient's eye and check this battery effect, we must test this voltage difference in an indirect manner, with the EOG. This is done by having the patient watch alternating lights from side-to-side, while an eye movement recording is being generated. The results of the eye movement recording are used to determine if the RPE is functioning normally.

# Preparing the Patient for an EOG

In order to record a valid EOG, the eye must be capable of being light-adapted sufficiently. In order to insure complete light adaptation, the eye must be dilated. After full dilation, five electrodes are placed on the patient's face. (A ground electrode is placed on the patient's forehead and four active electrodes are placed at the canthi of both eyes.) The skin must be cleaned with alcohol, taking care not to get the alcohol into the patient's eyes. Next, electrode paste is placed on the cleaned spots of skin and the electrodes are imbedded into the paste. Tape is used to secure the electrodes. Note Figure 7-1 for proper patient preparation.

# Recording the EOG

In order to record the voltage across the eye, the eye must rotate from one set of electrodes (the electrode at the lateral canthus of the left eye and the electrode of the medial canthus of the right eye) to the other (the electrode at the lateral canthus of the right eye and the electrode of the medial canthus of the left eye) (Figure 7-2).

Because the eyes actually move back and forth during the test one might assume that the width of the eye movements is directly related to the amount of right or left eye-swings. This is

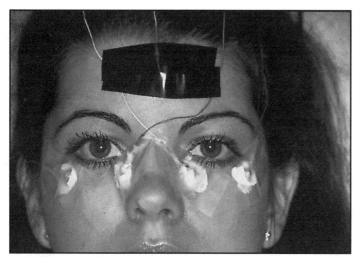

**Figure 7-1.** Patient prepared for EOG testing.

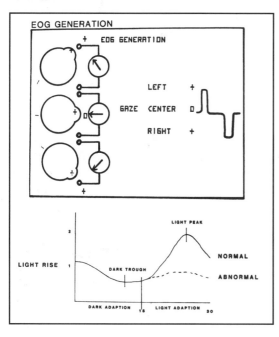

**Figure 7-2.** Representation of EOG eye movements. As the cornea moves to the right, the right electrodes will detect a positive charge as compared to the left electrodes and vice versa. The average of the eye movement amplitudes over time is illustrated below. After 15 minutes of dark adaptation, the eye movement amplitude becomes quite small. After 15 minutes of light adaptation, the eye movement amplitude becomes quite large in a normal individual, but remains small in those with generalized retinal and RPE cell abnormality. (Illustration courtesy of Thomas E. Ogden, MD, PhD.)

not the case. In actuality, the width of the eye movements (width of eye movement on a tracing) will actually get smaller in the dark and larger in the light from a normal eye (Figure 7-3).

If the eyes move back and forth but do not move to the target, then the eye movements will be random and therefore the test results will be meaningless. In order to eliminate this problem, the patient is asked to carefully watch the alternating diodes that are in the Ganzfeld bowl (the same bowl that is used for the ERG) (Figure 7-4) and to try not to move around much (Figure 7-5). If the patient watches the alternating diodes accurately, then the difference in the width of the eye movements is directly related to the change in voltage across the dark- and light-adapted eye (Figures 7-6 and 7-7). If the patient cannot watch the alternating diodes accurately (due to poor visual acuity, poor understanding of the test, or young age), then the width of the eye movements is meaningless and the test results are invalid (Figure 7-8).

**Figure 7-3.** A normal EOG as produced by a strip chart device. Most EOGs are done via computer, but not all computer programs produce actual eye movement tracings, as seen here. The two tracings on the left represent eye movements in the dark. The two tracings on the right represent eye movements in the light. The eye movements in the light should be about twice as large as those in the dark for normal individuals.

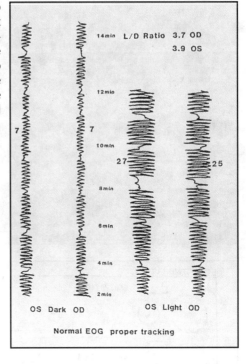

**Figure 7-4.** This is a view of the lighted Ganzfeld bowl. The left target light is lit, so the patient would look to the left. When the left light goes out, the right light will come on. The EOG is recorded by having the patient watch these alternating lights. (Reprinted with permission from Benes SC, McKinney K, Sanders LC, Miller M, Moberg M, *Advanced Ophthalmic Diagnostics and Therapeutics.* Thorofare, NJ: SLACK Incorporated; 1990.)

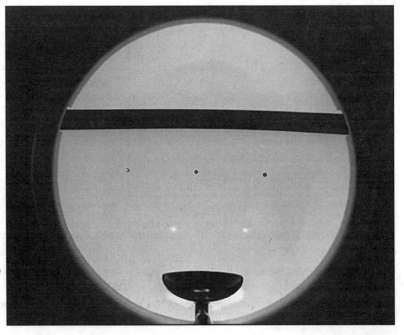

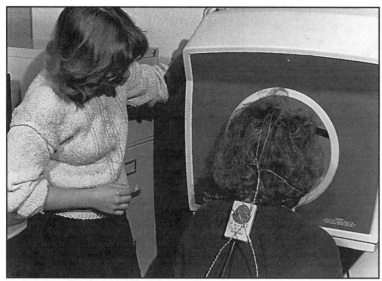

**Figure 7-5.** The patient sits forward and the chin is put in a centered chin rest in the Ganzfeld bowl. The patient is asked to remain perfectly still throughout the examination, since excessive movement renders the EOG invalid. (Reprinted with permission from Benes SC, McKinney K, Sanders LC, Miller M, Moberg M, *Advanced Ophthalmic Diagnostics and Therapeutics*. Thorofare, NJ: SLACK Incorporated; 1990.)

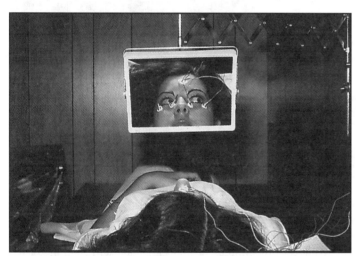

**Figure 7-6.** An illustration of proper eye movements necessary for EOG testing.

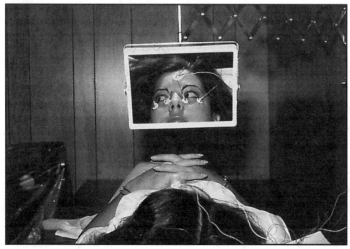

**Figure 7-7.** The patient looking in the opposite direction. Note the patient is supine and looking into a mirror. This was a common technique used in the past to insure proper head positioning. The use of the Ganzfeld bowl reduces a patient's ability to remain still for 30 minutes, thus reducing some of the reliability of the results. Exact eye movements, as seen in these two pictures, are essential for reliable EOG recordings.

**Figure 7-8.** An unreliable EOG tracing from a strip chart recorder. This represents poor fixation on the part of the patient which can be eliminated in many instances with proper coaching during the examination. Young children typically produce EOGs of this quality.

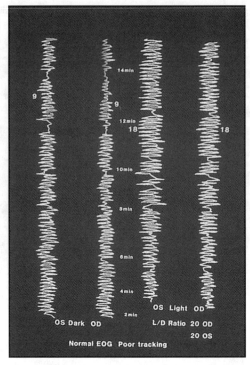

The patient is initially light-adapted for several minutes and then dark-adapted for 2 minutes. After the patient has been dark-adapted for 2 minutes (and while still in the dark) he or she is asked to watch the alternating diodes, usually for about 15 to 20 seconds. (The lights alternate about once every 2 seconds.) After the 15 seconds has lapsed and reliable eye movements have been recorded, the patient is asked to close his or her eyes. The patient will then be re-tested in a similar manner after 4 minutes, 6 minutes, 8 minutes, 10 minutes, 12 minutes, and 14 minutes of dark adaptation.

After the last dark-adapted eye movements have been recorded (at 14 minutes), the background light in the Ganzfeld bowl is turned on. After 2 minutes of light adaptation, the entire test procedure is repeated in the light. Instead of closing his or her eyes after the successful recording of eye movements, the patient is asked to stare straight ahead. The patient will keep his or her eyes open and staring straight ahead until the next recording session. The patient will then be re-tested at 4 minutes and every 2 minutes thereafter for 14 minutes, with his or her eyes open in between test sessions. This concludes the EOG test.

## What the Patient Needs to Know

- The EOG is not a painful test.
- It requires excellent cooperation, and you must remain as still as possible for the entire 30 minutes of the examination in order for a valid test to be recorded.
- If you cannot remain still, you should not undergo this type of testing.
- Your eyes will be dilated, so make proper transportation arrangements if necessary.
- The electrode paste and surgical tape can result in minor irritation in those with sensitive skin.

# Evaluating the EOG

The EOG tracing consists of numerous eye movements. The format of the EOG read-out is dependent on the type of equipment used. One type of unit produces an eye movement strip chart similar to the strip chart from an electrocardiogram. These tracings are easy to evaluate for quality and voltage change (see Figure 7-3). This type of unit produces the best EOG tracing, but is not used often. Most EOG read-outs are generated by a computer, and the computer provides information about the eye movement voltage (Figures 7-9 and 7-10). However in most situations, the examiner will need to calculate the voltage change from a dark-adapted to a light-adapted state (Figure 7-11).

The examiner must also evaluate the EOG recording for overall quality. Are the eye movements within each set fairly similar to one another, suggesting good fixation? Or is there significant variation within each test period? If the eye movements do not seem reliable within each test period then the test may be invalid, since it is likely that the patient did not fixate on the diodes accurately. If the eye movements seem reliable, then it is safe to evaluate the tracing. (See Figure 7-3 for a reliable EOG and Figure 7-8 for an unreliable EOG.)

The eye movement with the smallest amplitude in the dark is referred to as the "dark trough" (see Figure 7-3). The eye movement with the largest amplitude in the light is referred to as the "light peak" (see Figure 7-3). These values are then used to calculate the "Arden ratio" also known as the "light-peak/dark-trough" ratio (in which the light peak numeric value is divided by the dark trough numeric value.) This number is used to determine if the EOG falls within or outside of the normal range and whether the RPE cells are functioning normally or abnormally (see Figure 7-3 or Figure 7-11).

The dark trough and light peak eye movements are measured from peak-to-peak on one left-swing, right-swing sequence (Figure 7-12). On some units, the amplitudes of the dark trough and light peak are measured by the examiner (either with calipers or by the computer) and the Arden ratio is then calculated by hand. In some of the newer EOG units, both the dark trough and light peak voltages and the Arden ratio are calculated automatically by the computer. The computer plots the average of the eye movements of each test period, and then plots the averaged data.

The EOG findings represent a qualitative evaluation of how well the pigment epithelium and the rod photoreceptors are functioning. In most laboratories, an Arden ratio of 2.00 is well within the normal range, with the lower limits of normal being 1.70. Borderline normal EOGs are in the range of 1.69 to 1.56, and abnormal EOGs are virtually always below 1.55. Generally, patients with lighter fundi have higher Arden ratios than do those with darker fundi. Unlike the ERG, this test does not determine the percentage of involvement; it is purely qualitative. Normal Arden ratios generally indicate that the RPE is functioning normally, and abnormal ratios indicate that the RPE is functioning abnormally.

Some laboratories will set the upper range of abnormal at an Arden ratio higher than 1.55, such as 1.60. Each laboratory is encouraged to develop its own normative data. Slight variations in normal, borderline normal, and abnormal values are likely to be found between laboratories. EOG reports should indicate the normal, borderline normal, and abnormal ranges so that the EOG Arden ratios can be evaluated within the context of that particular laboratory's normal data.

Because the EOG requires patients to be cooperative, a normal Arden ratio is more significant than an abnormal Arden ratio. If the ratio is borderline normal or abnormal, it is important to establish the level of cooperation exhibited by the patient. If the patient was truly cooperative, did not close his or her eyes during the light adaptation portion, and did not move throughout the test,

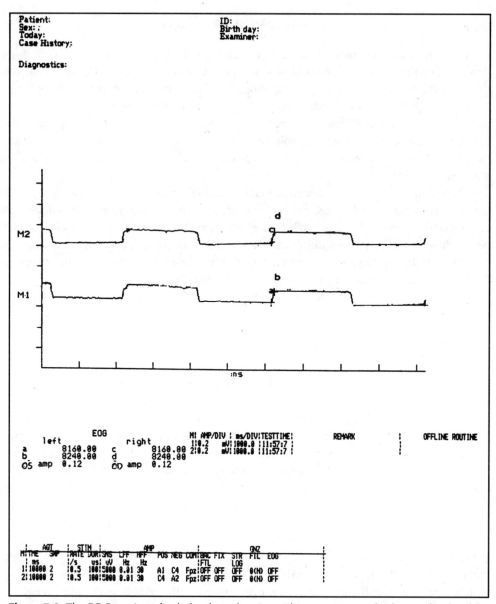

**Figure 7-9.** The EOG tracing of a dark-adapted patient. The examiner marks the amplitude of the eye movement by placing the cursor at each edge of the squared-off eye movement. The computer calculates the eye movement in microvolts. OD is represented by M2 and OS is represented by M1. The smallest amplitude represents the dark trough. (Reprinted with permission from Benes SC, McKinney K, Sanders LC, Miller M, Moberg M, *Advanced Ophthalmic Diagnostics and Therapeutics.* Thorofare, NJ: SLACK Incorporated; 1990.)

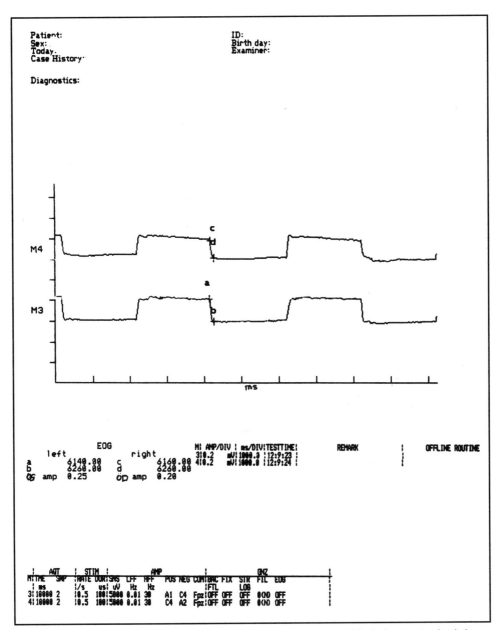

**Figure 7-10.** The EOG in a light-adapted state. There is a noticeable light rise in the left eye (M3) but less so in OD (M4). The eye movement amplitude is measured similarly to that noted in Figure 7-9. The largest amplitude represents the light peak. (Reprinted with permission from Benes SC, McKinney K, Sanders LC, Miller M, Moberg M, *Advanced Ophthalmic Diagnostics and Therapeutics.* Thorofare, NJ: SLACK Incorporated; 1990.)

Dear Dr.

Your patient _____ had an EOG

performed on ___8/18/87_____ .

The light peak was __0.25__ (mv ) OS ___0.20__ (mv·) OD.

The dark trough was _0.12__ (mv·) OS ___0.12__ (mv·) OD.

The Arden Ratio: $\frac{\text{light peak}}{\text{dark trough}}$ = __2.08__ OS __1.67__ OD

Normal values ≥ 1.75

Comments:___Normal EOG_____

_____

_____

_____

**Figure 7-11.** The EOG Arden ratio is calculated by taking the light peak and dividing it by the dark trough. The Arden ratio for OS is well within the normal limits at 2.08, but less than normal OD at 1.67. The ophthalmologist who analyzed the results felt that the low Arden ratio OD was due to artifact and interpreted the EOG as normal OU. This exemplifies the potential problems with using EOGs for diagnostic purposes. (Reprinted with permission from Benes SC, McKinney K, Sanders LC, Miller M, Moberg M, *Advanced Ophthalmic Diagnostics and Therapeutics.* Thorofare, NJ: SLACK Incorporated; 1990.)

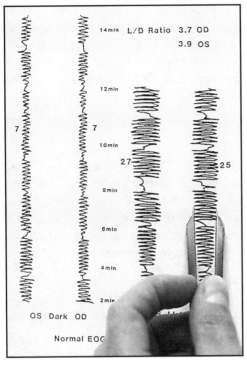

**Figure 7-12.** The EOG light/dark ratio can be measured by hand by measuring the smallest eye movement tracing from the dark phase (dark trough) and the largest eye movement tracing from the light phase (light peak). The amplitude of the light peak is divided by the dark trough amplitude to provide an Arden ratio (light/dark ratio). This computation is done by computer programs on most newer electrodiagnostic units. (Photograph by Nilo Davila.)

then the abnormal findings are likely to be significant. The borderline normal values (usually 1.60) are often the most difficult to evaluate, since the value could be due to insufficient light adaptation, early retinal and pigment epithelium pathology, or a variation of a normal value. Abnormal Arden ratios from a reliable EOG suggest that the RPE is functioning abnormally. The abnormal value is due to a lack of light rise during the light adaptation portion of the test. This lack suggests that the junctions between the pigment epithelium cells are not tight and a barrier between the two poles no longer exists. The EOG tracing in this scenario actually represents an eye movement test, where the amplitude of the eye movement is directly related to the right and left eye-swings and not related to the difference in voltage across the eye in either a dark- and light-adapted state. (This will become more obvious as we discuss the clinical usefulness of the EOG.)

## The Clinical Usefulness of the EOG

The EOG represents how well the RPE and rod photoreceptors are able to function. Thus the EOG is a useful test for any patient with a suspected retinal dystrophy. (I like to conduct EOGs on every patient with a suspected retinal abnormality since this data can support ERG findings, especially when the ERG findings are in the borderline normal range and the Arden value is in the abnormal range. With this scenario, a diagnosis of early retinal dystrophy can be easily made, for example.)

Some practitioners feel that the EOG is too unreliable (due to variabilities mentioned previously) and therefore should be used only on a limited basis. These practitioners generally use the EOG only if the person is suspected of having a disease the affects the pigment epithelium alone. Those who advocate such a position, however, probably do not obtain reliable EOGs on a regular basis. If the laboratories can produce reliable EOGs regularly, the usefulness of the test increases.

There are several disease processes in which the EOG is the diagnostic test of choice. These include Best's disease, other vitelliform macular dystrophies (the vitelliform lesion looks like an intact, yellow egg yoke directly on top of the macula), and early retinal toxicities (from either medications or intraocular metallic foreign bodies). A brief discussion of the EOG in severe retinal dystrophies will start this section, so that the concept of what the EOG is actually testing will be made clearer.

## The EOG in Retinitis Pigmentosa

The patient with end-stage retinitis pigmentosa has a virtually complete atrophy of both photoreceptor cells and pigment epithelium. EOGs in these patients are severely abnormal, with Arden ratios in the 1.00 and 1.30 range. Figure 7-13 is an example of a patient with end-stage retinitis pigmentosa. Note the virtual absence of light rise during the light adaptation phase. This example illustrates that if the RPE is absent from the eye, as in the case of end-stage retinitis pigmentosa, then the EOG will represent only eye movement and the "battery" effect is absent.

## The EOG in Best's Disease and Other Vitelliform Macular Dystrophies

Best's disease is an unusual juvenile-onset macular degeneration in which the ERG is normal and the EOG is abnormal. Onset of vision loss and funduscopic changes are usually found during the first two decades of life, but can also occur much later. In Best's disease, the pigment epithelium functions abnormally. Those individuals with Best's disease present with egg yoke-like lesions (vitelliform) in the posterior pole. They have a positive family history of macular degeneration as this is an autosomal dominant disease. Moreover, when tested, their ERGs will be normal and their EOGs will be abnormal. Individuals with Best's disease will generally have vision loss to the level of 20/200 and each of their offspring will have a 50% chance of inheriting the disease. (See Case History 7-1.)

Vitelliform lesions are also seen in other macular dystrophies. One such dystrophy is referred to as adult-onset vitelliform foveo-macular dystrophy of Gass. These individuals have reduced visual acuity, but only to the level of 20/70 or so. This is an autosomal recessive trait, so they will not likely pass this on to their offspring. The most significant difference between this disorder and Best's disease is that individuals with adult-onset vitelliform foveo-macular dystrophy of Gass have normal EOG findings. (See Case History 7-2.)

## The EOG in Retinal Toxicities Due to Medication

Certain medications can be toxic to both the retina and pigment epithelium. Systemic medications run throughout the bloodstream and eventually get to the place where the choroid interfaces with the RPE. The RPE acts as the blood/retina barrier designed to keep toxic medications from the delicate photoreceptor cells. If the medication is toxic to the RPE, the cells will eventually function abnormally and die off, thus reducing the effectiveness of the barrier. This can ultimately result in death to the photoreceptor cells if the patient is exposed to the medication for too long. In most instances, individuals will report eye problems prior to permanent loss of vision. However, using the EOG as a test of potential retinal toxicities may be helpful in early detection. (See Case History 7-3.)

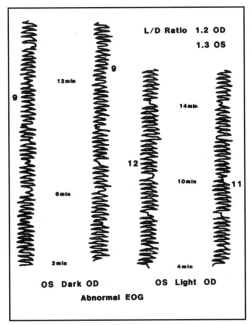

**Figure 7-13.** An abnormal EOG tracing from a strip chart recorder. Note the lack of light rise during the light adaptation phase. This is typical of patients with retinitis pigmentosa.

## The EOG in Retinal Toxicities Due to Retained Metallic Foreign Bodies

Metals such as iron can be extremely toxic to the retina. In some instances the EOG will be in the abnormal range prior to significant loss of photoreceptor cell function. This is particularly true if the metal has not been in the eye for a long period of time. Therefore, the EOG can be a useful test for detecting early retinal toxicities due to retained metallic foreign bodies. (See Case History 7-4.)

# Case Histories

## 7-1. Best's Disease

The patient was a 13-year-old female with a history of sudden onset vision loss. She was found to have an egg-yoke type lesion in one eye, and the other eye had a macular scar.

She underwent ERG and EOG testing and was found to have a normal ERG and an abnormal EOG of 1.2 OD and 1.3 OS. She was thus diagnosed with Best's disease.

Because this is an autosomal dominant disorder, one of her parents also had to have the disease. It was found that her maternal grandfather had been treated for age-related macular degeneration. When tested with both the ERG and EOG, he was found to have a normal ERG and an abnormal EOG of 1.1 OD and 1.2 OS. Thus he, too, had Best's disease, although his symptoms occurred when he was old enough to be diagnosed with run-of-the-mill macular degeneration.

The girl's mother had to be the "missing link" between the grandfather and granddaughter. The mother's funduscopic examination was unremarkable in both eyes, but her EOG was abnormal at 1.3 OD and 1.4 OS. Although the mother had no funduscopic changes, it is likely that she will develop macular degeneration at a later date. The gene that causes Best's disease does not affect every individual in the same way, as can be seen in this example. The EOG was a helpful adjunct to clinical findings.

## 7-2. Adult-Onset Vitelliform Foveo-Macular Dystrophy of Gass

The patient was a 43-year-old female with a history of mildly reduced visual acuity of 20/40 in each eye. She presented with vitelliform lesions in both eyes and a provisional diagnosis of Best's disease.

She underwent both an ERG and EOG. Both tests were normal; the EOG Arden ratios were 1.7 OD and 1.8 OS. These results were not consistent with Best's disease, but rather with adult-onset vitelliform foveo-macular dystrophy of Gass (most of those affected have low, but normal Arden ratios.) Her visual prognosis is significantly better than it would be if she had Best's disease, and she will not have to worry that her children inherited her eye problems.

## 7-3. Plaquenil Toxicity

The patient was a 17-year-old female who had a history of taking Plaquenil (Sanofi Pharmaceuticals Inc., New York, NY) (which has a slight chance of causing retinal toxicity) to control symptoms associated with rheumatoid arthritis.

She was tested with an EOG prior to being started on the medication. Her Arden values were within the normal range at 2.2 OD and 2.1 OS. About 1 year later, she started noticing some subtle changes in her color vision. She went to her ophthalmologist and was found to have normal funduscopic findings in both eyes. She underwent EOG testing again. This time the Arden ratios were 1.6 OD and 1.5 OS. The right eye was in the borderline normal range, but the left eye was clearly abnormal. Her ERG was normal in both eyes.

She was taken off the Plaquenil and re-tested about 6 months later. On follow-up, her Arden ratios were 1.9 OD and 2.0 OS, again in the normal range. She reported that her color vision also had returned to normal.

## 7-4. Retinal Toxicity From a Retained Metallic Foreign Body

The patient was a 47-year-old male who had a history of metallic intraocular foreign body in the right eye. He underwent vitrectomy and his retinal surgeon felt that the metal had been completely removed. To verify this, the ophthalmologist ordered an ERG and EOG about one month postoperatively.

The ERG of the right eye was mildly reduced in amplitude, but within the normal range. The EOG was clearly abnormal with an Arden ratio of 1.4. The very mild reduction in ERG amplitude was felt to be due to the surgery, but the clearly abnormal EOG could not be explained. The patient was suspected to have a retained (but unseen) metallic foreign body.

The patient was asked to come back in 3 weeks for a repeat ERG and EOG. On repeat testing, the EOG was again abnormal, but this time the ERG was clearly abnormal in the right eye, confirming that there was a retained metallic foreign body. The patient underwent a second vitrectomy and additional metal was found and removed.

The patient was re-tested about 6 months postoperatively, at which time the Arden ratio was within the normal range at 1.7. The ERG amplitude was improved in the right eye, but did not recover to the level of the fellow eye, suggesting that there was permanent damage to the photoreceptor cells due to prolonged exposure to the metallic foreign body.

# Chapter 8

# Visual Evoked Response

### KEY POINTS

- The visual evoked response (VER) is a response by the brain to a visual stimulus.

- The flash VER is the best overall test to determine how well the visual system is functioning.

- The pattern VER can only be recorded if the patient reliably watches the stimulus.

# Introduction to the Visual Evoked Response

The visual evoked response (VER), also known as the visual evoked potential (VEP) or visual evoked cortical potential (VECP), is a brain response to specific visual stimuli. The test is somewhat similar to an electroencephalogram (EEG) in which random brain waves are detected by tiny electrodes placed on the patient's scalp. In the EEG, all areas of the brain are tested and the recording represents continuous brain activity over time. The VER is also an electrode-detected brain wave test but it is a test of a certain area of the brain known as the visual or occipital cortex.

The visual cortex is located at the back of the head in both hemispheres of the brain. Unlike the EEG, the VER is an evoked response, meaning that the visual stimulus causes the brain to respond. The main purpose of obtaining a VER is to determine how well the visual system of the individual is functioning. The VER provides excellent information about the functional integrity of the visual system, and is the best overall test to determine how well the visual system works. The test can show whether the visual system works well in general, works poorly, or does not work at all.

A disadvantage of the VER is that it does not indicate which part of the visual system is abnormal. Thus, an individual may have a dense corneal leukoma, retinal detachment, compressed optic nerve, or tumor in the visual cortex. Any of these very different abnormalities will produce similarly abnormal VER results. Although this test may not provide all of the information that may be desired, using it along with the ERG and EOG can provide useful information about the integrity of the visual system. It can provide useful diagnostic information as well.

# Stimuli

There are three basic types of stimuli that can be used to evoke the visual response from the visual cortex. These include a flashing light, an alternating checkerboard pattern, and a moving sinusoidal grating of varying frequencies and contrasts.

For most ophthalmic VERs, both a flashing light stimulus and an alternating checkerboard pattern stimulus are used (Figures 8-1 and 8-2). The response from the flashing light provides information about the basic integrity of the visual system and can be used on virtually any patient, including crying or uncooperative ones. The response from the alternating checkerboard pattern provides general information about visual acuity, and patients must cooperate by watching the pattern in order for a response to be recorded.

The moving sinusoidal grating is frequently employed in laboratory settings. This pattern has been used to evaluate visual development in human infants, and also requires patient cooperation. The brain waves generated by these different visual stimuli look remarkably different. This will be discussed in detail later.

# Averaging

In the EEG, brain activity is recorded on one continuous strip for a period of 30 minutes or so. This means of recording shows random brain activity over time. Normal brain activity can produce both very large brain waves (that can be as large as 100 µv in amplitude) and very small brain waves.

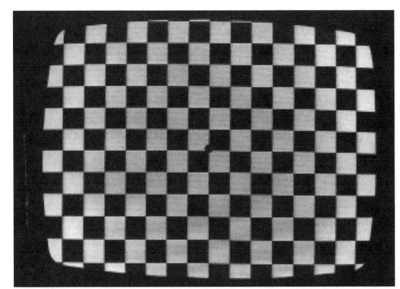

**Figure 8-1.** An alternating checkerboard pattern used for pattern VER testing. (Reprinted with permission from Benes SC, McKinney K, Sanders LC, Miller M, Moberg M, *Advanced Ophthalmic Diagnostics and Therapeutics*. Thorofare, NJ: SLACK Incorporated; 1990.)

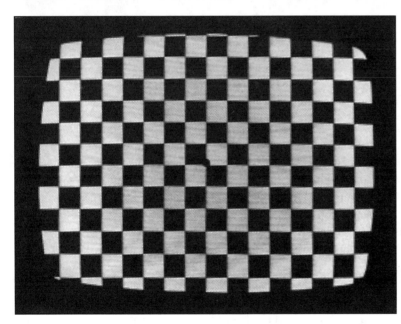

**Figure 8-2.** The checks alternating between black and white and white and black as depicted in this figure and Figure 8-1. The rate of alternation can be changed by the examiner, but are generally presented to the patient at approximately two full alternations per second. (Reprinted with permission from Benes SC, McKinney K, Sanders LC, Miller M, Moberg M, *Advanced Ophthalmic Diagnostics and Therapeutics*. Thorofare, NJ: SLACK Incorporated; 1990.)

The VER is a test of brain activity that does not look at random brain activity over time, but is concerned with specific brain activity over a limited period of time. Put another way, the VER represents visual cortex activity from the time a stimulus is shown (in this case, from the time the light flashes) until about a half second after the light has flashed. This is the amount of time it takes the eye to respond to the light and send a signal to the brain.

If the eye were exposed to a single flash of light, for instance, the recorded waveform would include the response of the visual cortex to the visual stimulus as well as random brain activity. The response would look similar to an EEG. This is because the response of the visual cortex to the visual stimulus is small in amplitude at 10 μv or so, but the random brain activity might be as large as 100 μv. Therefore, the visual response would be "covered up" by the random brain activity.

In order to eliminate this problem, the VER is averaged. Instead of flashing a single light in the patient's eye, the examiner will test the patient repeatedly up to 200 times. The responses are then combined within the computer (this process is known as averaging) to produce a VER. The responses are not laid end-to-end, but are superimposed on one another. This can be done because the brain response to the visual stimulus is time-locked to that stimulus. In most individuals, the brain's response to a visual stimulus occurs at about 100 msecs (one-tenth of a second) after the flash of light. This response does not change. For instance, if a patient has a response at 105 msecs, then no matter how many times the patient views the stimulus (assuming that the intensity of the light and the distance of the light from the patient remain the same), the response will be generated by the brain at 105 msecs. This is what is meant by a response being time-locked to the stimulus.

Random brain activity is just that—random. On any one brain wave tracing there may be a large amplitude response at 75 msecs one time and a very small response at the same location the next time. After the individual has been exposed to the flashing light about 100 times, a robust visual evoked response remains, but most of the random brain activity will have been removed by means of averaging (Figure 8-3). Averaging is done regardless of the type of stimulus used during testing.

# VER Testing

## Preparing the Patient

Several electrodes are placed on the patient's scalp. Unlike the EEG, only one active electrode is placed on the scalp (in most clinical settings) one centimeter above the occipital protuberance in the midline position. (In other words, the electrode is placed about a half inch above the little bump on the back of the head, in a position that is equidistant from both ears. You can probably find your own occipital protuberance by feeling for the bump on the back of your head.) The electrode is placed in the midline position so that both hemispheres of the brain can be tested simultaneously. (Both hemispheres can be tested separately, requiring three active electrodes on the scalp; one over the left visual cortex, one in the midline position, and one over the right visual cortex.)

Before the electrode can be placed on the patient's head, the scalp must be prepared. First, part the hair so that the scalp can be seen. Second, find the location where the electrode should be placed. Next, wipe the scalp with isopropyl alcohol and an abrasive paste such as Omni-Prep. (This is to ensure good contact between the electrode and the scalp.) Next, wipe off the excess abrasive paste; the scalp should be quite clean at this point. Place a ½ inch ribbon of electrode paste, such as EC-2 cream, on the clean area of scalp. Place the electrode in the paste and secure with several pieces of tape. The same procedure is used for cleaning and attaching two additional electrodes, a reference electrode (usually on the top of the head in a midline position) and a ground electrode (usually placed on the forehead) (Figures 8-4 through 8-6).

The impedance of each electrode must be checked. Impedance is a numeric value that suggests whether the electrode has made good contact with the skin or scalp (low impedance) or has made bad contact with the skin or scalp (high impedance). Low impedance suggests that the electrode has made good electrical contact and that electrical activity from the brain will be easily recorded. The impedance can be measured using the electrophysiology unit, or with a hand-held

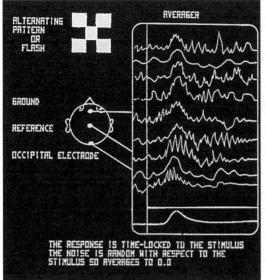

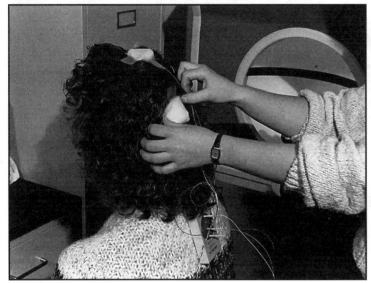

**Figure 8-3.** Each time the patient is stimulated by the flash a small visual response is recorded. But this response is so small that brain "noise" virtually eliminates it from view. Numerous responses are averaged where brain noise is averaged away, leaving a robust VER. (Reprinted with permission from Van Boemel GB, Ogden TE. Clinical Electrophysiology. In: Ryan SJ, ed. *Retina.* St. Louis, Mo: Mosby-Year Book; 1999.)

**Figure 8-4.** The active electrode is placed 1 cm above the occipital protuberance in the midline position. The reference electrode is placed on the crown of the head, also in the midline position. The cotton helps keep the electrodes in place. (Reprinted with permission from Benes SC, McKinney K, Sanders LC, Miller M, Moberg M, *Advanced Ophthalmic Diagnostics and Therapeutics.* Thorofare, NJ: SLACK Incorporated; 1990.)

**Figure 8-5.** The ground electrode is placed on the forehead in the midline position. Electrodes are secured with surgical tape. (Reprinted with permission from Benes SC, McKinney K, Sanders LC, Miller M, Moberg M, *Advanced Ophthalmic Diagnostics and Therapeutics.* Thorofare, NJ: SLACK Incorporated; 1990.)

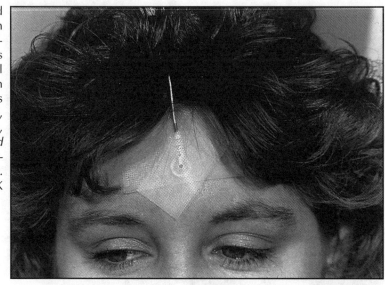

**Figure 8-6.** The electrodes are secured in the pre-amplifier (attached to the patient's collar) that is connected to the computer. The non-tested eye is patched with a gaze eye pad and black electrical tape to insure that the non-tested eye is not inadvertently tested. (Reprinted with permission from Benes SC, McKinney K, Sanders LC, Miller M, Moberg M, *Advanced Ophthalmic Diagnostics and Therapeutics.* Thorofare, NJ: SLACK Incorporated; 1990.)

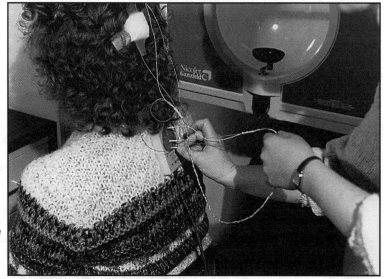

impedance meter. If the impedance is high, then the electrode should be removed and the skin cleaned again. Impedance values should be less than 5. Higher numbers suggest poor contact and poor impedance. Poor impedance can result in very noisy and unreliable tracings.

Each eye must be tested separately. The untested eye should be adequately occluded to insure that no light enters it accidentally; this is usually accomplished by covering the untested eye with an eye pad and opaque tape (such as electrical or pipe tape). The patient is now ready for VER testing.

## Administering the Test

International standards have not yet been set for VER testing, though it is likely that there will be (for the practice of ophthalmology) at some time in the future. In general, the patient is first

## What the Patient Needs to Know

- (Prior to the test) Bring your glasses.

- You will not be dilated for the examination.

- Make sure your hair is clean (although you will need to wash it again after the test). This is not the time for a fancy hairdo.

- (During the test) The VER is not a painful test and generally takes less than 45 minutes.

- Electrodes will be placed on your head. The skin and scalp will need to be cleansed prior to electrode placement. The cleansing of the skin and scalp requires rubbing, and this may be uncomfortable for some individuals.

- Now and then, patients will have a temporary headache after the test. Take a regular pain reliever if your headache persists.

- If you have epilepsy, please tell us. In rare cases the flashing light can trigger a seizure.

- You will need to wear your glasses for part of the test.

- After the test has been completed, the electrodes will have to be removed. The tape may pull on your hair or skin.

- There will be residual electrode paste left on the scalp after the electrodes are removed. Wash your hair when you get home. The electrode paste comes out easily with soap and warm water.

tested by looking at a flashing light that is presented successively for 100 repetitions. (The technician needs to note whether the patient has a history of epilepsy. If so, the flashing light stimulus will need to be presented to the patient manually in a random fashion.) The patient watches the flashing light from within the Ganzfeld bowl. A complex waveform should result from this type of stimulation (see Figures 8-9 through 8-13 for examples of normal flash VERs). After a reliable tracing has been recorded, a second tracing is recorded to verify the response. The VER tracing is repeated because brain noise and VERs can look surprisingly similar. By repeating the VER two or three times, a reproducible response can be obtained (Figure 8-7). If the response is not reproducible, then it is likely that the patient has a non-recordable flash VER, since the brain activity that has been recorded is probably random brain noise (Figure 8-8).

After the patient has undergone the flash VER, he or she will be tested with the alternating checkerboard pattern VER (see Figures 8-1 and 8-2). First, the patient is set at a predetermined distance from the television monitor and asked to wear his or her best correction. (The patient's eyes should not be dilated.) The patient is then shown the smallest checkerboard pattern and a response is recorded. In most testing situations, the checkerboard alternates 100 times until a visual evoked response is visible. A second response, using the same size pattern, is obtained to ensure that the response is real and not random brain activity.

If a reproducible response is obtained, the examiner will next show the patient the largest checkerboard and record at least 2 responses. This will provide information about how quickly the brain responds to visual stimuli. (The response can be abnormal in visual pathway conduc-

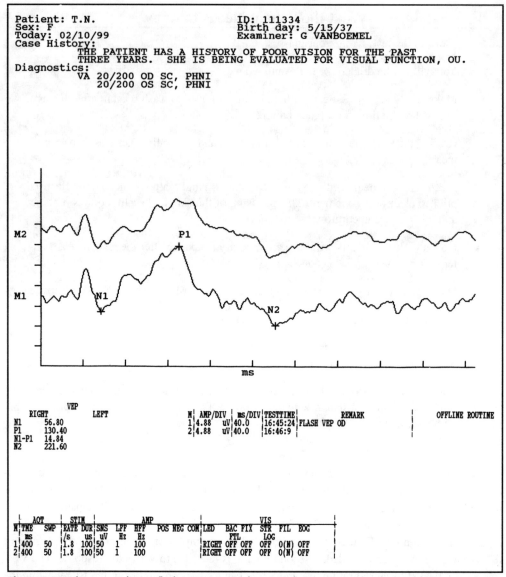

Patient: T.N.                              ID: 111334
Sex: F                                     Birth day: 5/15/37
Today: 02/10/99                            Examiner: G VANBOEMEL
Case History:
              THE PATIENT HAS A HISTORY OF POOR VISION FOR THE PAST
              THREE YEARS.  SHE IS BEING EVALUATED FOR VISUAL FUNCTION, OU.
Diagnostics:
              VA  20/200 OD SC, PHNI
                  20/200 OS SC, PHNI

VEP

| | RIGHT | LEFT | | N | AMP/DIV | ms/DIV | TESTTIME | REMARK | | OFFLINE ROUTINE |
|---|---|---|---|---|---|---|---|---|---|---|
| N1 | 56.80 | | | 1 | 4.88 uV | 40.0 | 16:45:24 | FLASH VEP OD | | |
| P1 | 130.40 | | | 2 | 4.88 uV | 40.0 | 16:46:9 | | | |
| N1-P1 | 14.84 | | | | | | | | | |
| N2 | 221.60 | | | | | | | | | |

| | AOT | | STIM | | | AMP | | | | | VIS | | | |
|---|---|---|---|---|---|---|---|---|---|---|---|---|---|---|
| N | TIME | SWP | RATE | DUR | SNS | LFF | HFF | POS | NEG | COM | LED | BAC | FIX | STR | FIL | EOG |
| | ms | | /s | us | uV | Hz | Hz | | | | | | FTL | LOG | | |
| 1 | 400 | 50 | 1.8 | 100 | 50 | 1 | 100 | | | | RIGHT | OFF | OFF | OFF | O(N) | OFF |
| 2 | 400 | 50 | 1.8 | 100 | 50 | 1 | 100 | | | | RIGHT | OFF | OFF | OFF | O(N) | OFF |

**Figure 8-7.** When recording a flash VER, a complex waveform, as seen here, should become visible. Two VERs should be recorded for each stimulus used. This eliminates the possibility of mistaking brain noise for a response. The bottom tracing was recorded first. The second tracing looks somewhat different than the first. This may be due to unequal illumination (such as from the eye closing during the second recording). If the two recordings look any different than this (depicted here), there should be a third response recorded.

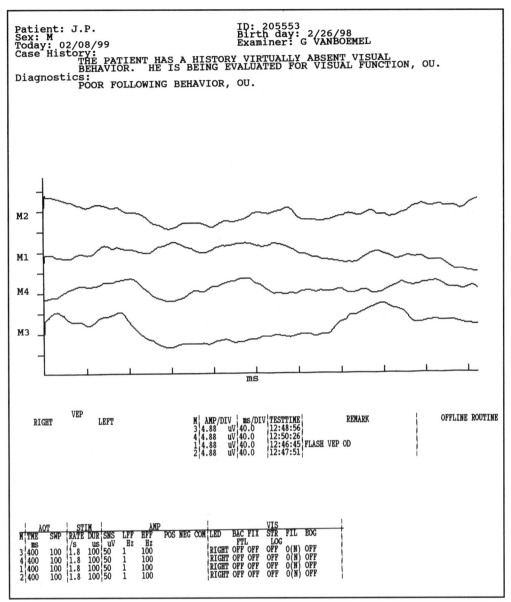

Patient: J.P.
Sex: M
Today: 02/08/99
Case History:
THE PATIENT HAS A HISTORY VIRTUALLY ABSENT VISUAL
BEHAVIOR. HE IS BEING EVALUATED FOR VISUAL FUNCTION, OU.
Diagnostics:
POOR FOLLOWING BEHAVIOR, OU.

ID: 205553
Birth day: 2/26/98
Examiner: G VANBOEMEL

M2

M1

M4

M3

ms

VEP
RIGHT          LEFT

| N | AMP/DIV | ms/DIV | TESTTIME | REMARK | | OFFLINE ROUTINE |
|---|---------|--------|----------|--------|---|---|
| 3 | 4.88 uV | 40.0 | 12:48:56 | | | |
| 4 | 4.88 uV | 40.0 | 12:50:26 | | | |
| 1 | 4.88 uV | 40.0 | 12:46:45 | FLASH VEP OD | | |
| 2 | 4.88 uV | 40.0 | 12:47:51 | | | |

| N | AOT | | STIM | | | AMP | | | | VIS | | | |
|---|-----|-----|------|-----|-----|-----|-----|-----|-----|-----|-----|-----|-----|
| | TIME ms | SWP | RATE /s | DUR us | SNS uV | LFF Hz | HFF Hz | POS | NEG | CON | LED | BAC FIX FTL | STR LOG | FIL | EOG |
| 3 | 400 | 100 | 1.8 | 100 | 50 | 1 | 100 | | | | RIGHT | OFF OFF | OFF | O(N) | OFF |
| 4 | 400 | 100 | 1.8 | 100 | 50 | 1 | 100 | | | | RIGHT | OFF OFF | OFF | O(N) | OFF |
| 1 | 400 | 100 | 1.8 | 100 | 50 | 1 | 100 | | | | RIGHT | OFF OFF | OFF | O(N) | OFF |
| 2 | 400 | 100 | 1.8 | 100 | 50 | 1 | 100 | | | | RIGHT | OFF OFF | OFF | O(N) | OFF |

**Figure 8-8.** Brain noise can frequently look like a response, as can be observed in this non-recordable flash VER. The bottom two flash VERs look somewhat like a small and abnormal response, but repeated testing shows that the "response" cannot be reproduced each time. Differentiating small responses from brain noise is particularly important when trying to evaluate visual potential in individuals with very poor vision.

tion abnormalities such as optic neuritis.) If the patient does not respond to the smallest checkerboard pattern, he or she is shown the next larger pattern, and so on, until two identical responses can be obtained from the same-sized checkerboard pattern. If the patient does not respond to any checkerboard pattern, then he or she either has severely reduced visual acuity (generally worse than 20/400) or has not watched the checkerboard pattern well enough for a response to be generated by the brain. After testing the patient with the alternating checkerboard pattern, the patch is moved so that the other eye can be evaluated by the same process.

# Evaluating Test Results

## The Flash VER Waveform

The normal flash VER consists of a complex pattern that is present in the first half of the waveform. (The flash VER waveform generally has a 400 to 500 msecs duration, thus one should find a complex pattern within the first 200 to 250 msecs.) This complex pattern contains a large positive peak (a waveform that has a peak above the baseline) at approximately 100 msecs from the time of the flash known as P1 or P100, immediately preceded by a negative peak (a waveform that has a peak below the baseline) at approximately 90 msecs from the time of the flash (N1 or N100). A normal flash VER should have the following four characteristics: a complex set of waveforms that include an N1 and P1 waveform, a P1 waveform that is 5 μv in amplitude or greater within the first 250 msecs, no delay in the P1 peak (primary wave), and symmetry between the two eyes.

As indicated, there are several key waveforms that should be present in the normal flash VER. The first is the P1 or P100 waveform. The P2 or P200 is the second positive waveform at approximately 200 msecs. The N1 or N100 is the first negative waveform and the N2 or N200 is the second negative waveform at approximately 200 msecs. Figure 8-9 shows the typical "M" and Figure 8-10 shows the typical "W" shaped pattern associated with a normal flash VER tracing. Note the P1, P2, N1, and N2 waveforms.

The waveform that is of greatest importance is the P1 waveform. The P1 amplitude (or height) is measured from the trough of the N1 waveform to the peak of the P1 waveform. The amplitude is generally calculated by the computer and shown in the computer printout (Figure 8-10). The amplitude of the normal P1 waveform should be 5 μv or greater. A P1 amplitude of 3 μv or less is generally considered abnormal in most laboratories.

The peak delay of the P1 waveform is also important. The peak delay is calculated as the time from the onset of the stimulus to the peak of the P1 waveform. The peak delay of the P1 waveform is generally 100 msecs (one-tenth of a second). The peak delay represents how quickly the brain responds to the visual stimulus. This information is also calculated by the computer and included in the printout (see Figure 8-10).

Unlike the ERG (which is fairly similar between individuals), variability in VER waveforms is quite common, as can be seen by the great variety of normal VER tracings in this section. This variation occurs because other brain activity contributes to the VER, and such things as head size and skull density can also affect this cortical response (Figures 8-11 through 8-13). However, there are several types of abnormalities that can be noted in flash VER findings. First, low amplitude responses that are not complex in waveform are often abnormal. In many laboratories the P1 waveform must be at least 3 μv in amplitude to be considered normal. However, some individuals with normal visual systems can have very small VER amplitudes. This can be due to bone density of the skull and other factors such as poor cooperation or electrode displacement.

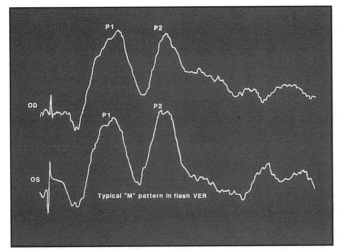

**Figure 8-9.** A typical "M" shaped flash VER. The examiner looks for a complex waveform in the first half of the sweep as noted here.

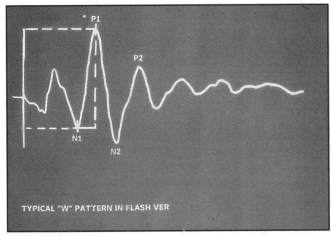

**Figure 8-10.** There are several important waves that should be observed in a normal flash VER. They include the N1, P1, N2, and P2, The most important wave is the P1, wave that should be located at about 100 msecs from the onset of the flash and should be a least 4 µv in order to be considered normal. The amplitude of the P1 wave is measured from the trough of the N1 to the peak of the P1. The latency of the P1 waveform is measured from the onset of the stimulus to the peak of the P1 wave.

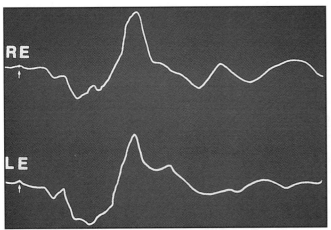

**Figure 8-11.** There is significant variability noted in normal VER waveforms. However, the responses from the two eyes should be symmetric, as seen here. (Illustration courtesy of Thomas E. Ogden, MD, PhD.)

**Figure 8-12.** Some have distinct N1, P1, N2, and P2 waves. (Illustration courtesy of Thomas E. Ogden, MD, PhD.)

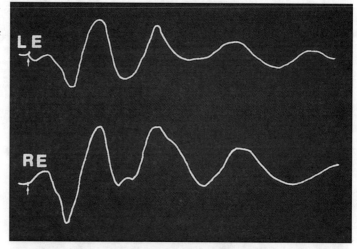

**Figure 8-13.** Some have only N1 and P1 waves. (Illustration courtesy of Thomas E. Ogden, MD, PhD.)

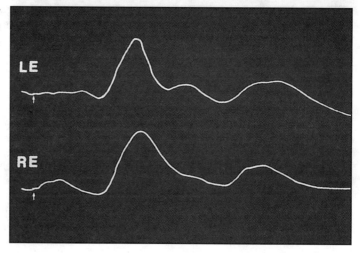

Prolongation of P1 peak delay can also represent a visual pathway abnormality. In most laboratories, the P1 is at 100 msecs and is still considered to be in the normal range at 120 msecs. Most electrophysiologists would agree that the P1 is delayed at 130 msecs. Delay in the P1 waveform can be consistent with such disorders as optic neuritis and other visual pathway abnormalities. When evaluating the flash VER waveform, there should be less than 10% variability between the two eyes in both peak delay and amplitude. Variability of over 25% is considered significant for pathology. Abnormality in VER waveforms can thus be more easily detected if only one eye is affected (Figure 8-14).

If the two waveforms do not look the same, then the waveform that fits the "typical pattern" of the flash VER is probably normal. The flash VER that is reduced in amplitude, slow, or "simplified" (a term used to denote a waveform that has very few negative and positive peaks, or one that looks similar to the normal fellow eye, but looks smoothed out) is probably abnormal (see Figure 8-14).

Unfortunately, just because the waveforms look significantly different from one another does not mean that it is easy to determine which eye is abnormal. Therefore, it is important to obtain a thorough history on individuals who are undergoing VER testing to know which eye is affect-

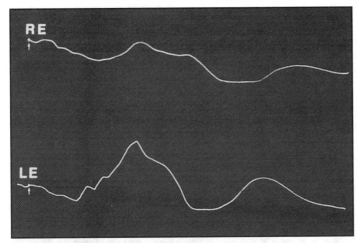

**Figure 8-14.** Asymmetry, as noted in this picture, suggests some type of pathology, either at the level of the retina or the central visual pathways, from the affected eye. The response from the right eye has a lower amplitude, is abnormal, and is easily recognized. (Illustration courtesy of Thomas E. Ogden, MD, PhD.)

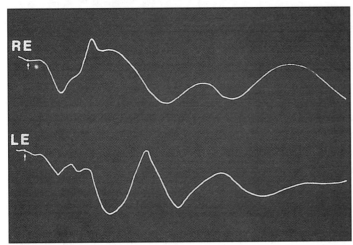

**Figure 8-15.** There is obvious asymmetry noted here, but determining which eye is abnormal is more difficult. The left eye appears to be the one with the abnormal VER, but, in fact, it is the right that is abnormal. (Illustration courtesy of Thomas E. Ogden, MD, PhD.)

ed. As seen in Figure 8-15, it is not easy to determine which tracing is abnormal when both are complex but look very different from one another. The tracing from the right eye in this figure is abnormal, although that tracing might not be the one you would suspect. The examiner was aware that the right was the abnormal eye by talking with the patient. That information was used to determine which flash VER was normal and which was abnormal. Viewing the flash VER without supporting documentation about the patient's complaints would have made it virtually impossible to determine that the VER from the right eye was abnormal.

## The Pattern VER Waveform

The pattern VER waveform is much less complex than that of the flash VER. The pattern VER waveform consists of a single-peaked response at approximately 100 msecs (P1 or P100). There are generally very few other waveforms noted on the response, and the response between individuals is quite similar (unlike that of the flash VER).

The presence of the pattern VER is very significant because the pattern VER can help establish approximate visual acuity in individuals who cannot provide accurate verbal responses. The pattern VER can also be used to determine if a demyelinating process is present (such as optic

**Figure 8-16.** The pattern VER waveform consists of a single P1 or P100 wave, as seen here. Note the normal pattern VER tracing from the same eye using various check sizes. The check size is indicated by the Snellen equivalent noted on the right. (Smaller checks correspond to better Snellen acuities.) Responses to smaller checks are lower in amplitude and somewhat delayed, as compared to responses to larger checks (as seen here). A robust response to certain checks indicates objective visual acuity. The VER on the bottom is from a flash stimulus. (Illustration courtesy of Thomas E. Ogden, MD, PhD.)

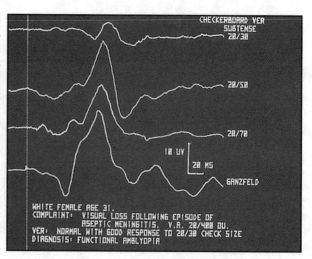

neuritis). Optic neuritis can be diagnosed if there is a prolongation of the P1 peak delay. The absence of a pattern VER is not as significant, as the patient must be able to see the alternating checkerboard pattern clearly in order for a response to be generated. Individuals who have very poor vision, who are uncooperative, or who have uncorrected refractive errors will not have responses to the checkerboard pattern.

In most laboratories, the patient is tested with the smallest check first and then the next largest check until a reproducible response is obtained as noted earlier. The patient is always tested with one of the larger checks in order to determine the peak delay of the pattern VER response (Figure 8-16). The peak delay is measured from the stimulus artifact to the peak of the P1 waveform (see Figure 8-16). The peak delay of the response to the largest check should not be prolonged, and a P1 response of over 120 msecs is considered abnormal. The amplitude of the waveform is not considered as critical, since P1 amplitudes can decrease when the patient does not adequately fixate on the checkerboard pattern. The amplitude is measured from the onset of the P1 waveform to the peak of the P1 waveform (see Figure 8-16).

Prolongation in pattern VER peak delay is very important and generally indicates some type of visual pathway abnormality (frequently associated with conduction problems, as in optic neuritis). The peak delay of the waveform should be the same between the two eyes; any asymmetry greater than 5 msecs would be considered significant even if the peak delay of the prolonged waveform was under 120 msecs.

The only way that a pattern VER can be obtained is if the person adequately watches the pattern. This is because the alternating checks must fall on the retina and must result in a sharp and clear image. If the patient blinks excessively or does not look directly at the pattern, the image will not fall on the retina (Figure 8-17). If the patient has an uncorrected refractive error or reduced visual acuity, the image will not be sharp and clear (Figure 8-18). Obviously then, there are many reasons why a pattern VER may not be recordable. A non-recordable pattern VER may not be consistent with widespread ocular pathology, but may be more consistent with poor patient cooperation. It is essential that patient cooperation be noted when this test is performed, especially when evaluating a non-recordable pattern VER.

A recordable pattern VER, on the other hand, is very significant and can reveal that a person who is describing severely reduced visual acuity has, in fact, much better acuity than claimed. Some laboratories have collected pattern VER data from reliable individuals with various levels

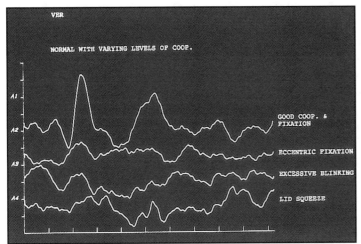

**Figure 8-17.** Pattern VER testing requires excellent fixation. Note the top pattern VER response and the large P1 waveform. Poor fixation, excessive blinking, and lid squeezing eliminates the response. (Illustration courtesy of Deidre Martin, University of California, Los Angeles.)

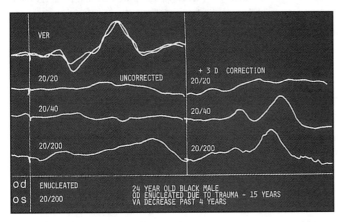

**Figure 8-18.** Pattern VER testing requires that the patient be properly refracted. Note the virtual absence of pattern response on the left and the robust response on the right that is present after the patient is refracted. The response is from the left eye, as the right eye has been enucleated.

of vision loss to be able to correlate pattern VER results with actual visual acuity. These labs may frequently be asked to estimate a patient's visual acuity from a VER. The visual acuity is usually estimated at a 95% confidence level, since there is always the remote possibility that a person actually has worse or better vision than the pattern VER test estimates (this can be true especially if the patient has irregularities of the cornea, as in keratoconus).

The VER can thus be used to estimate visual acuity in individuals who are malingering, who may have a psychogenic component to the unexplained vision loss, who are pre-verbal (such as infants), or who are non-verbal (such as individuals with dementia). However, these types of individuals may also be prone to uncooperative behavior, so any non-recordable pattern VER results must be interpreted with caution. In this type of situation, noting cooperation level is especially critical.

## The Clinical Usefulness of Flash and Pattern VER Testing

Both the flash and pattern VER can be extremely useful in assessing visual function in individuals with ocular disease. The responses to the two types of visual stimuli provide different information about visual system integrity, so both types of tests are generally done on each patient. (In some situations only flash VER testing is done, but in the majority of cases, both the flash and pattern VER are recorded.)

There are several key situations in which VER testing should be conducted. These include evaluating individuals with unexplained vision loss (either organic or non-organic), evaluating visual potential (as in non-verbal infants), assessing optic nerve disease, evaluating or determining visual cortex abnormality, and determining retinal versus visual pathway abnormality. These situations will be discussed in detail below.

## Evaluation of Unexplained Vision Loss

As many as 7% of all individuals who are seen in an ophthalmology clinic have vision loss that may be classified as unexplained. In some instances there is a non-organic component to the claim, such as an individual who is feigning vision loss to obtain monetary compensation through a lawsuit. Others with unexplained vision loss might have a severe psychological problem that results in a non-organic vision loss. Finally, an individual may have a previously undiagnosed cortical abnormality that results in vision loss that is not easily explained. The VER can be a helpful adjunct to the regular eye examination when evaluating individuals with unexplained vision loss. (Please see Case Histories 8-1 through 8-4.)

## Evaluation of Visual Potential

There are times when it is difficult to assess a patient's visual potential. This is particularly true in individuals who are pre-verbal, non-verbal, or who have poorly documented histories and ocular findings. The VER can be helpful in assessing vision in such cases. A normal VER can offset the fears of parents whose child does not seem to be seeing well. (See Case History 8-5.)

Depending on where you work, it is possible that you will see patients who have had very little eyecare in the past. In such cases, it may be difficult to adequately assess visual potential. If the patient presents with a dense cataract and a history that may include closed angle glaucoma or trauma, then determining visual potential prior to surgery may be helpful. A flash VER can be useful in such an evaluation. (See Case Histories 8-6 and 8-7.)

## Evaluation of Optic Nerve Disease

The VER can be a useful diagnostic tool when assessing optic nerve disease. This is particularly true in the case of optic neuritis. In patients with optic neuritis, the P1 waveform is significantly delayed. This is true for both the flash and pattern VER, but is especially true for the pattern VER. That is why it is necessary to record a pattern VER with large check sizes, since large check sizes produce the shortest P1 peak delays. (See Case History 8-8.)

## Evaluation of Visual Cortex Abnormality

Evaluation of cortical blindness has already been discussed in this section under the heading of evaluating unexplained vision loss. In some instances, cortical blindness is initially suspected after an insult such as stroke, head trauma, or anoxia. (See Case History 8-9.)

### Differentiation of Retinal Versus Visual Pathway Abnormalities

When an individual presents with profound loss of vision and the underlying etiology is unclear, both the ERG and the VER are used to determine the location of the abnormality. There are some instances when the history itself leads to a conclusion regarding the underlying etiology. Other times the history can imply either retinal or cortical abnormality as the underlying cause of vision loss. This is the situation when obtaining both an ERG and VER is essential. (See Case History 8-10.)

# Case Histories

## 8-1. Unexplained Vision Loss From a Possible Malingerer

The patient was a 59-year-old female who had a history of being splashed in the face with battery acid 2 years before. At the time of the accident she was sent to the emergency room and the acid was adequately rinsed from her eyes. She had no residual corneal scarring. She reported that her vision deteriorated during the 2 years following the incident, and she presented with hand-motion vision in both eyes. There was a lawsuit pending.

Her VER was recorded. The tracing in Figure 8-19 reveals a normal flash VER in both eyes. Note the robust P1 waveforms. The patient also had a pattern VER response to a very small check size, subtending an angle of arc of less than 5 minutes. Therefore, her vision is significantly better than hand-motion, as she retains excellent form vision. (In my laboratory, we would report that her vision was better than 20/30 in both eyes at a 95% confidence level, based on these findings.) If she truly had hand-motion vision, her pattern VER would have been nonrecordable even when tested with very large checks. It is likely that the individual was malingering.

## 8-2. Unexplained Vision Loss With a Probable Psychological Etiology

The patient was a 9-year-old female who had normal vision and normal health prior to visiting her father for 2 months. Upon her return home, she complained of significant gastrointestinal problems, headaches, insomnia, and severely reduced vision to the level of 20/200 OD and 20/ 100 OS. She had undergone a full physical examination by a family practitioner who found no physical problems to account for her poor health. An ophthalmologist also examined her and found no physical findings to account for her profound loss of vision in both eyes. She was sent for VER testing to rule out cortical blindness.

Her VER was recorded. The tracing in Figure 8-20 reveals a normal flash VER in both eyes. Note the robust P1 waveforms. This patient had a pattern VER response to a very small check size, subtending an angle of arc of less than 5 minutes. This suggests that her vision was significantly better than claimed, probably along the lines of 20/30 or better in both eyes at a 95% confidence level.

This young patient probably had a psychogenic component to explain her vision loss. In other words, she was probably hysterically blind. This can be substantiated by the fact that she had other profound health problems that are not based on organic pathology. (There is a psychiatric

**Figure 8-19.** Flash and pattern VER testing can be a helpful when trying to assess whether a patient has organic pathology to account for vision loss. This patient had battery acid splashed in her face, without residual corneal scarring. Her vision deteriorated over a period of 2 years and she was thought to be malingering. She claimed hand-motions vision in both eyes, but her pattern VER results suggest vision better than 20/20, OU. This patient was probably malingering. (Illustration courtesy of Thomas E. Ogden, MD, PhD.)

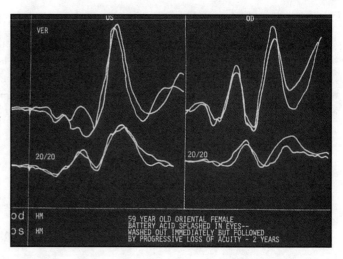

disorder, called somatization disorder, that results in numerous health complaints such as severe headaches, profound vision loss, dizziness, non-specific pain, and gastrointestinal problems of non-organic etiology.)

It is possible that the child was a victim of some type of trauma, either physical or psychological, that occurred while she was in the care of her father. This type of patient should undergo a full psychological work-up to determine if there is a history of trauma or conflict that has resulted in her health and visual complaints.

## 8-3. Unexplained Vision Loss, Provisional Diagnosis: Malingering

(Author's note: This is a case history from a patient I saw in the mid-1980s. I do not see patients like this anymore, but this is an excellent example of how useful a VER can be in determining cortical abnormalities in individuals who are suspected of malingering.)

The patient was a 49-year-old male with a 7-month history of reduced visual acuity. His ocular findings were normal; however, he had numerous health complaints including cowpox and neurosyphilis. He had been relatively healthy prior to the onset of his vision loss. He reported that everything looked "odd" to him.

His VER was recorded. His cooperation level was excellent. The tracing in Figure 8-21 reveals a severely abnormal flash VER in both eyes. Note the poorly developed response and low amplitude P1 waveforms. This patient had no pattern VER responses, even to the largest check sizes. The pattern VER findings were consistent with his reported visual acuity.

A report was sent to his attending ophthalmologist who sent the patient on to neurology because of the abnormal flash VER findings. The patient was found to have herpetic encephalitis secondary to AIDS (acquired immune defiency syndrome), which had been undiagnosed prior to his VER testing. Thus, the VER revealed significant pathology that resulted in further work-up and ultimate diagnosis for this unfortunate patient.

*Author's note:* At that time there were no blood tests to detect HIV (human immunodefiency virus), and doctors were reluctant to give a patient such a diagnosis because treatment modalities were so poor. Today, it is unlikely that a patient would be that ill without knowing the underlying etiology causing such profound symptoms.

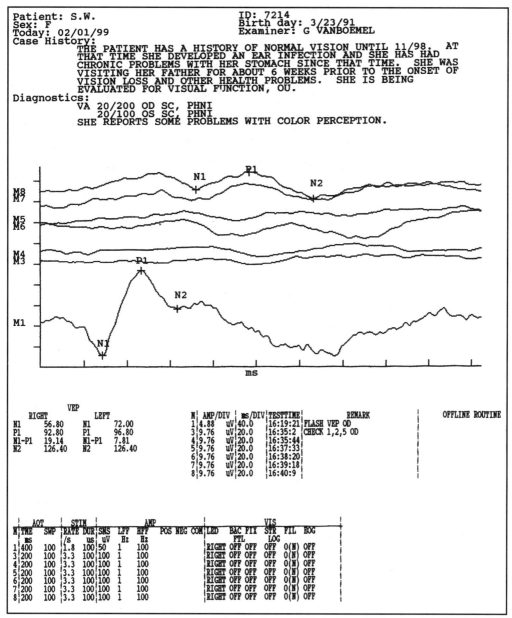

**Figure 8-20.** This VER was recorded from a 9-year-old girl who had visited her estranged father for 6 weeks. Prior to going to visit him, she was perfectly normal. Upon her return, she had severely reduced visual acuity and numerous health complaints that could not be explained by medical examination and were felt to be non-organic. Her claimed visual acuity was 20/200 OD and 20/100 OS, but her pattern VER findings suggested vision of better than 20/30, OU. Note the small but reproducible response with the smallest check (M3 and M4). (Check responses are displayed at 50% of normal.) This compilation of findings could be consistent with psychogenic blindness.

**Figure 8-21.** This VER was recorded from a man who was thought to be malingering. Note the very low and abnormal amplitude from the flash VER and the non-recordable pattern VER. The patient was later found to have herpetic encephalitis as a result of AIDS. (Reprinted with permission from Van Boemel GB, Ogden TE. Clinical Electrophysiology. In: Ryan SJ, ed. *Retina*. St. Louis, Mo: Mosby-Year Book; 1999.)

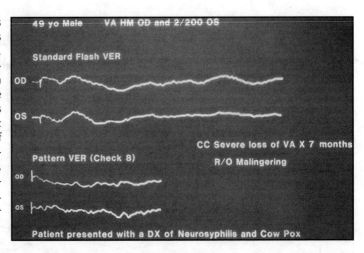

## 8-4. Unexplained Vision Loss, Provisional Diagnosis: Malingering

The patient was a 60-year-old male with a 7-year history of no light perception in both eyes. He had undergone brain surgery involving the visual cortex area 7 years ago, and upon recovering from the surgery had no light perception vision. He insisted that he could see things, although his wife knew that he could not. She had applied for blind disability benefits for him, which required that he undergo a full ophthalmologic examination. The eye exam was unremarkable; he had normally reactive pupils. He was referred for VER testing with a provisional diagnosis of malingering.

His VER was recorded. His cooperation level was excellent. The tracing in Figure 8-22 reveals a non-recordable flash VER in both eyes. Note the absence of P1 waveforms. This patient had no pattern VER responses, either.

This patient's diagnosis was determined to be cortical blindness and not malingering. The normal reaction of the pupils would be consistent with cortical blindness, since the pupillary fibers go back as far as the lateral geniculate and not all the way to the visual cortex. The patient's insistence that he can "see" is also consistent with cortical blindness, where the eye and primary cortex are often normal. Information thus gets to some part of the brain, but is not processed properly. The original diagnosis of malingering was used in part because of his normal eye findings and in part because he was applying for monetary compensation for his vision loss.

## 8-5. Poor Visual Behavior in an Otherwise Healthy Baby

The patient was a 6-month-old female who presented with nystagmus and very poor visual behavior. Her ocular findings were normal. She was sent for VER testing to determine visual potential and rule out cortical blindness.

Her VER was recorded. The tracing in Figure 8-23 reveals a normal flash VER in both eyes. Note the robust P1 waveforms. This patient also had a pattern VER response to a large check size. This suggests that the patient has at least some form vision, although she may not have normal 20/20 acuity. Testing indicated that her vision was better than 20/200 in both eyes at a 95% confidence level. (An ERG was also normal, see Figure 6-30.)

Although it is impossible to determine what this child's ultimate visual acuity may be, the VER conveys to both the ophthalmologist and the parents that the child has some useable vision,

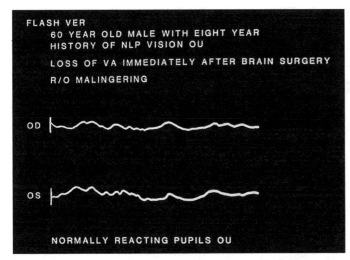

FLASH VER
60 YEAR OLD MALE WITH EIGHT YEAR
HISTORY OF NLP VISION OU

LOSS OF VA IMMEDIATELY AFTER BRAIN SURGERY

R/O MALINGERING

OD

OS

NORMALLY REACTING PUPILS OU

**Figure 8-22.** This flash VER was recorded from a man who was also thought to be malingering. He had undergone brain surgery in the area of the visual cortex and reported NLP vision after the surgery. He had normally reactive pupils, OU. His non-recordable flash VER findings support his claims of NLP vision and a diagnosis of cortical blindness.

regardless of poor visual behavior. This could be consistent with delayed visual maturation, where an infant's visual behavior develops more slowly than expected.

## 8-6. Presence of Dense Cataract and Unknown Ocular History

The patient was a 39-year-old male with a history of trauma to the right eye with subsequent traumatic cataract. The patient did not obtain adequate eyecare after the injury. He was being evaluated for visual potential in his previously injured right eye. His visual acuity was measured as hand motions OD and 20/20 OS.

His VER was recorded. The tracing in Figure 8-24 reveals a normal flash VER in both eyes. Note the robust P1 waveforms. These findings would suggest that he has good visual potential in the previously traumatized eye. While there is no guarantee of the post-operative visual acuity, there is an adequate VER response to justify taking out the cataract in the right eye.

## 8-7. Presence of Dense Cataract and Unknown Ocular History

The patient was a 30-year-old male with a history of trauma to the right eye, with subsequent corneal scar and traumatic cataract. He did not obtain adequate eyecare after the injury. He reported experiencing excessive pain in the right eye, associated with nausea at the time of injury. After several days he went to the hospital and was found to have closed-angle glaucoma. He was currently being evaluated for visual potential prior to possible cataract extraction and penetrating keratoplasty in his previously injured right eye. Visual acuity was measured as 20/20 OS and light perception OD.

His VER was recorded. The tracing in Figure 8-25 reveals a normal flash VER in the non-injured eye, but a severely abnormal flash VER in the injured eye. Note the severe reduction of the P1 waveform from the injured eye. These findings would suggest that he has very little visual potential in the right eye. Ocular surgery would not improve the visual acuity in the right eye beyond that of his reported light perception vision; therefore surgery would not be indicated.

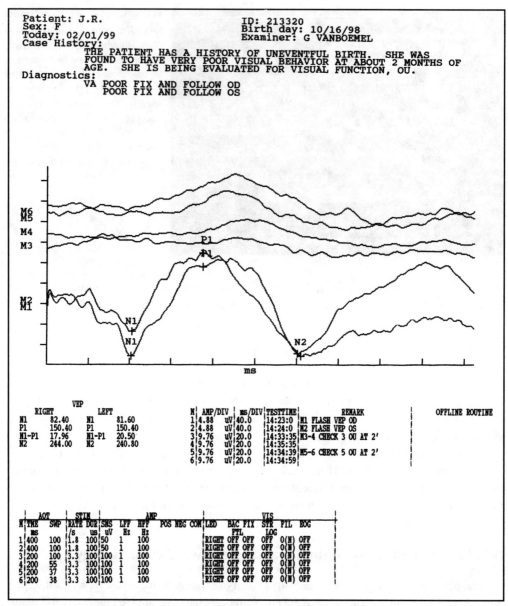

Patient: J.R.
Sex: F
Today: 02/01/99
Case History:
    THE PATIENT HAS A HISTORY OF UNEVENTFUL BIRTH.  SHE WAS
    FOUND TO HAVE VERY POOR VISUAL BEHAVIOR AT ABOUT 2 MONTHS OF
    AGE.  SHE IS BEING EVALUATED FOR VISUAL FUNCTION, OU.
Diagnostics:
    VA POOR FIX AND FOLLOW OD
    POOR FIX AND FOLLOW OS

ID: 213320
Birth day: 10/16/98
Examiner: G VANBOEMEL

**Figure 8-23.** A normal flash (bottom two tracings) and pattern VER from a 6-month-old child with virtually absent visual behavior. Her ERG was also normal (see Figure 6-30). These findings are consistent with delayed visual maturation. Her vision should eventually become normal.

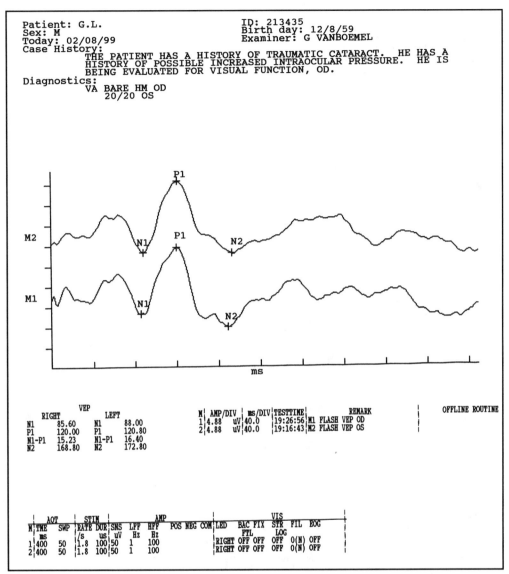

```
Patient: G.L.                    ID: 213435
Sex: M                           Birth day: 12/8/59
Today: 02/08/99                  Examiner: G VANBOEMEL
Case History:
        THE PATIENT HAS A HISTORY OF TRAUMATIC CATARACT.  HE HAS A
        HISTORY OF POSSIBLE INCREASED INTRAOCULAR PRESSURE.  HE IS
        BEING EVALUATED FOR VISUAL FUNCTION, OD.
Diagnostics:
        VA BARE HM OD
           20/20 OS
```

```
                        VEP
        RIGHT         LEFT            N  AMP/DIV   ms/DIV TESTTIME           REMARK              OFFLINE ROUTINE
N1      85.60    N1    88.00          1  4.88  uV  40.0   19:26:56 M1 FLASH VEP OD
P1      120.00   P1    120.80         2  4.88  uV  40.0   19:16:43 M2 FLASH VEP OS
N1-P1   15.23    N1-P1 16.40
N2      168.80   N2    172.80
```

```
       AOT      STIM            AMP                          VIS
N  TIME  SWP  RATE DUR SNS LFF HFF  POS NEG CON LED  BAC FIX STR FIL EOG
   ms         /s   us  uV  Hz  Hz                    FTL     LOG
1  400    50   1.8 100 50  1   100              RIGHT OFF OFF OFF O(N) OFF
2  400    50   1.8 100 50  1   100              RIGHT OFF OFF OFF O(N) OFF
```

**Figure 8-24.** Flash VER testing can be used to determine if a patient should undergo surgery to remove media opacities, such as corneal scars or dense cataracts. This patient presented with a dense traumatic cataract and there were concerns that he might have had elevated intraocular pressure at one time. The flash VER is normal and symmetric, thus suggesting good visual potential from an eye claiming bare hand-motions vision.

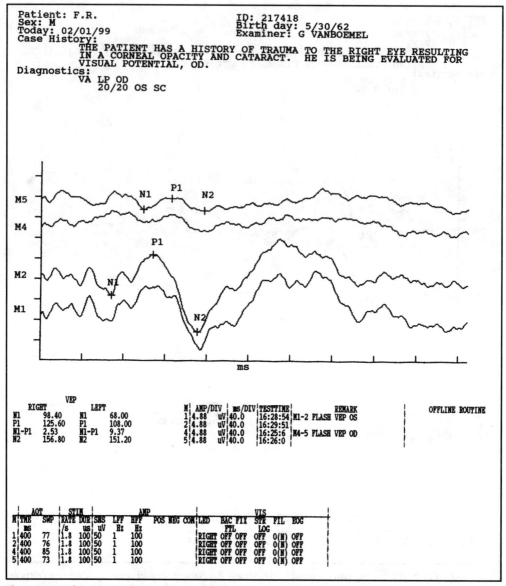

**Figure 8-25.** This patient also presented with an eye with a traumatic cataract, corneal opacity, and light perception vision, OD. These results suggest a different visual prognosis, however. Note the severely abnormal response from the right eye (top two tracings), suggesting very poor visual potential.

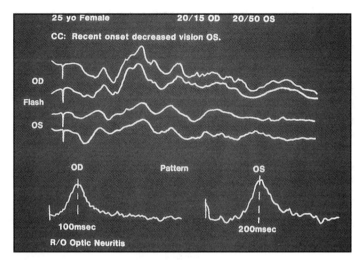

**Figure 8-26.** Flash and pattern VER testing can be used for detecting early optic neuritis. The pattern VER is especially helpful, as a prolongation of latency signals a conduction abnormality along the optic nerve. The flash VER from the left eye is reduced in amplitude and slightly slowed, but the P1 latency of the pattern response from the left eye is clearly abnormal at 200 msecs. The normal eye had a latency of 100 msecs.

## 8-8. Probable Optic Neuritis

The patient was a 25-year-old female with history of sudden loss of vision in the left eye. She complained of blurred vision and poor color perception, OS. Her visual acuity was 20/20 OD and 20/50 OS. She went to her ophthalmologist who noted no significant eye findings, but suspected that she had optic neuritis in the left eye. He ordered VER testing.

Her VER was recorded. The tracing in Figure 8-26 reveals a normal flash VER in the right eye, but an abnormal response from the left eye. Note the poorly developed and delayed P1 waveform OS as compared with OD. The pattern VER at the largest check size revealed a normal peak delay OD and a severely prolonged peak delay (200 msecs) OS. These findings for the left eye are consistent with a diagnosis of optic neuritis, in which the P1 peak delay is always prolonged.

## 8-9. Cortical Blindness Due to Anoxic Encephalopathy

The patient was a 5-year-old female with a history of anoxic encephalopathy due to cardiac arrest during an emergency appendectomy. Upon recovery her vision was severally reduced to 20/200 OD and 2/200 OS; her funduscopic examination was unremarkable. She was sent for a VER with a tentative diagnosis of cortical blindness.

Her VER was recorded. The tracing in Figure 8-27 reveals a severely abnormal and symmetric flash VER. Note the virtual absence of P1 waveforms from both eyes. The absence of the P1 waveform is significant, since this represents visual cortex functioning. The results are consistent with a diagnosis of cortical blindness.

## 8-10. Radiation Retinopathy Versus Cortical Blindness Due to Radiation

The patient was a 26-year-old male with a history of brain tumor for which he underwent full head radiation. Several months after radiation he reported a marked loss of visual acuity in both eyes to the level of hand motions, OU. He presented with mild retinal hemorrhages. It was suspected that radiation retinopathy was responsible for his light perception vision in both eyes. He underwent both ERG and VER testing to confirm the diagnosis.

**Figure 8-27.** Flash VER testing can be used to detect cortical blindness. A complex waveform should be noted at about 100 msecs. This is a VER from a 5-year-old child who went into cardiac arrest during an emergency appendectomy resulting in anoxic encephalopathy. She has a very abnormal flash VER, with virtual absence of a P1 waveform.

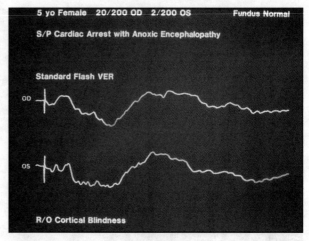

His ERG was recorded and revealed a mild reduction in b-wave amplitude, with associated mild slowing. His VER was also recorded, and was barely recordable (not depicted). These results reveal that, although there were retinal changes in both eyes, the underlying etiology of profound vision loss was not due to radiation retinopathy, but rather to cortical blindness as a result of full head radiation.

# Bibliography

Apple DJ, Rabb MF. *Ocular Pathology: Clinical Applications and Self-Assessment.* St. Louis, Mo: Mosby Year Book; 1991.

Benes SC, McKinney K, Sanders LC, Miller M, Moberg M. *Advanced Ophthalmic Diagnostics and Therapeutics.* Thorofare, NJ: SLACK Incorporated; 1990.

Burkitt HG, Young B, Daniels VG. *Wheater s Functional Histology: A Text and Color Atlas.* Edinburgh, Scotland: Churchill Livingstone; 1993.

Burton GRW, Engelkirk EG. *Microbiology for the Health Sciences.* Philadelphia, Pa: JB Lippincott Co; 1996.

Byrne SF, Green RL. *Ultrasound of the Eye and Orbit.* St. Louis, Mo: Mosby Year Book; 1992.

Carr RE, Siegel IM. *Electrodiagnostic Testing of the Visual System: A Clinical Guide.* Philadelphia, Pa: FA Davis Co; 1990.

Colenbrander A. Principles of ophthalmology. In: Tasman W, Jaeger EA, eds. *Duane s Ophthalmology on CD-ROM.* Philadelphia, Pa: Lippincott-Raven Publishers; 1996.

Davis BD, Dulbecco R, Eisen HN, Ginsberg HS. *Microbiology.* 4th ed. Philadelphia, Pa: JB Lippincott Co; 1990.

Engelberg AL, ed. *Guides to the Evaluation of Permanent Impairment.* 3rd ed. Philadelphia, Pa: American Medical Association; 1988.

Fishman GA, Sokol S. *Electrophysiologic Testing in Disorders of the Retina, Optic Nerve, and Visual Pathway.* San Francisco, Calif: American Academy of Ophthalmology; 1990.

Gass JDM. *Stereoscopic Atlas of Macular Diseases: Diagnosis and Treatment.* St. Louis, Mo: CV Mosby Co; 1987.

Green RL, Bryne SF. Diagnostic ophthalmic ultrasound. In: Ryan SJ, ed. *Retina.* St. Louis, Mo: CV Mosby Co; 1989.

Jimenez-Sierra JM, Ogden TE, Van Boemel GB. *Inherited Retinal Diseases: A Diagnostic Guide.* St. Louis, Mo: CV Mosby Co; 1989.

Kendall CJ. *Ophthalmic Echography.* Thorofare, NJ: SLACK Incorporated; 1990.

Koneman EW, Allen SD, Dowell VR, Janda WM, Sommers HM, Winn WC. *Color Atlas and Textbook of Diagnostic Microbiology.* 3rd ed. Philadelphia, Pa: JB Lippincott Co;1988.

Nadler MP, Miller D, Nadler DJ, eds. *Glare and Contrast Sensitivity for Clinicians.* New York, NY: Springer-Verlag; 1990.

Stein HA, Slatt BJ, Stein RM. *The Ophthalmic Assistant.* 5th ed. St. Louis, Mo: CV Mosby Co; 1988.

Vaughan DG, Asbury T, Riordan-Eva P. *General Ophthalmology.* 13th ed. Norwalk, Conn: Appleton & Lange; 1992.

# Disability Determination: Who Qualifies and Who Doesn't

`LV`

**KEY POINTS**

- In the United States, individuals with visual acuity of 20/200 or worse in the better eye after correction are considered legally blind.

- Individuals with significant visual field loss, where the greatest width of the field is 20 degrees or less in the better eye, are also considered legally blind.

- Individuals who are legally blind are entitled to certain benefits such as monetary compensation, free or reduced cost public transportation, free telephone services, and other free services specifically designed for the blind.

In a perfect world, every patient who comes in for eyecare would have an easily treatable disease and would always regain 20/20 visual acuity after our interventions. Unfortunately, such a scenario does not exist. For those individuals with permanent vision loss, proper documentation and disclosure may result in improved living. Eyecare physicians might not discuss the patient's reduced visual acuity or might maintain that the patient's vision may, in fact, improve. Such lack of disclosure can result in the patient not seeking benefits to which he or she is entitled. The patient may also think that his or her poor vision is not considered disabling. Allowing patients the opportunity to understand their level of vision loss may result in their feeling more at ease, and may result in their seeking services to which they are entitled. A frank discussion with each visually impaired patient would be advised. Helping the patient understand the definition of legal blindness and what such a definition implies may also be an important part of the patient/physician/technician interaction.

## Impairment and Disability

In order for an individual to be considered disabled, that individual must have an impairment. An impairment is a physical change in a person's health status that is evaluated by a physician and described in medical terms. Disability is assessed in non-medical terms and is used to indicate that a person is unable to meet social, personal, or occupational demands. In other words, impairment is what is physically or mentally wrong with the patient, while disability connotes the difference between what a person wants to do and what that individual is able to do because of the presence of the physical or mental impairment. In ophthalmology, physical impairment is based on eye disease; disability is based on how the vision loss reduces the person's ability to work and recreate. If a person has an impairment, it does not always imply that he or she is disabled. For instance, a person who has been employed as a transcriptionist may not be disabled by macular degeneration, whereas a person who has been employed as an accountant may be extremely disabled by the same condition. A person is considered disabled only after the impairment has resulted in a change in functioning in that individual.

## Definitions of Vision Loss

`OptT`

There are different definitions of vision loss; however, most definitions are designed to convey level of disability that is present based on vision loss. The World Health Organization (WHO) has designated visual impairment categories to be used for documenting vision loss. They include: moderate visual impairment with vision ranging from 20/70 to 20/160 in the better eye after correction; severe visual impairment with vision ranging from 20/200 to 20/400 in the better eye after correction, or visual fields that subtend an angle of arc of no greater than 20 degrees; profound visual impairment with vision ranging from 20/500 and 20/1000 in the better eye after correction, or visual fields that subtend an angle of arc of 10 degrees or less; near-total visual impairment with vision ranging from worse than 20/1000 to light perception in the better eye after correction, or visual fields that subtend an angle of arc of 5 degrees or less; and total visual impairment with vision at the no light perception level.

The World Health Organization categorization of vision loss is used in the International Code of Diseases (ICD). In the United States, the term "legal blindness" is used to denote vision loss that is considered disabling. Legal blindness has been defined as vision loss of 20/200 or worse

`OptA`

in the better eye after correction, a visual field of 10 degrees or less from central fixation in the better eye, or a visual field that subtends an angle of arc of 20 degrees or less. Such definitions are relatively arbitrary; however, those who do not meet these strict guidelines may still be considered disabled, as will be discussed later in this section.

# Importance of Determining Level of Impairment and Disability

Determining the level of impairment may be very important, since many individuals who are legally blind may not be able to work. Moreover, those individuals who are not legally blind but have serious eye conditions may be considered disabled, also. In such cases, these disabled individuals may be compensated monetarily, either through insurance and social service programs such as Worker's Compensation or Social Security. Moreover, the legally blind individual may be eligible for free or reduced fee services such as public transportation and large-size telephones. Legally blind individuals can obtain free material through the Library of Congress and can take a special deduction on their income taxes. Legally blind individuals may be eligible for handicap parking plaques as well.

The federal registry also recognizes that many individuals who are not legally blind may be disabled based on vision loss. Persons who have total bilateral ophthalmoplegia, complete bilateral homonymous hemianopsia, or reduced visual efficiency (based on reduced visual acuity and constricted visual fields) may also be eligible for certain benefits. Such benefits should be available to all who qualify, but many people will not know that they qualify without sufficient disclosure from the ophthalmologist and his or her staff.

On the other hand, a person should not be considered legally blind unless there is sufficient documentation to support the classification. The American Medical Association (AMA) suggests that each physician follow the same procedures when making such a classification, so that a second physician would come to the same conclusion about the patient being evaluated. Therefore, a classification of legal blindness should not be given to a patient who has vision of 20/200 or worse in the better eye unless there is clinical evidence to support such vision loss.

## Assessing and Documenting Vision Loss

In order to document vision loss, it should be assessed in a standardized manner so that virtually the same results and conclusions can be drawn by a second examiner. Visual disabilities can be based on reduced central acuity, constriction of visual fields, a combination of visual field and central acuity loss, other conditions (such as ophthalmoplegia), or mild vision loss in combination with other physical impairments.

### Central Visual Acuity

Central visual acuity should be documented at both distance and near with and without standard correction (not low vision correction or contact lens correction) by means of a standardized vision chart such as a Snellen chart. Test chart illumination for distance vision testing should be at least 5 foot-candles. This lighting allows for about an 85% contrast of the vision chart. The test distance of 20 feet is used to simulate infinity. A shorter distance can be used to simulate infinity, but no shorter than 13 feet. When testing at near, a near Snellen, Jaeger, or American point-type chart can be used. If a non-Snellen near chart is used, one must be mindful of the conversion from Jaeger or point readings to Snellen equivalents. Standard correction and distance of about 13 inches should be used for the near measurement, and the chart should be illuminated with an overhead lamp that is about three times brighter than the room light. Visual acuity should be documented (for both distance and near, with and without correction) in the patient's chart. Any variation from the standard procedure should be documented also.

Vision loss at both distance and near corresponds to specific percentages of loss. Tables A-1a and A-1b illustrate the percentage of loss at both distance and near. In many instances, the person's distance and near vision is about the same. However, if that is not the case, a combined percentage that takes the average of both distance and near vision can be calculated (Table A-2). For instance, the average value for an 80% loss of vision at near and a 60% reduction at distance results in a 70% overall reduction of vision.

Generally speaking, vision loss is considered disabling if it represents an 80% loss of visual function in both eyes. However, certain circumstances besides visual acuity may actually increase the percentage of vision loss. If the patient is monocularly aphakic or pseudophakic, there is an additional loss of vision in addition to that calculated by near and distance vision. For example, suppose a person who is not aphakic has a combined vision loss equal to an 80% reduction of vision. A person with similar vision who is monocularly aphakic will have a 90% reduction of vision. The impairment of being monocularly aphakic is weighted by an additional 50% loss of the remaining vision. (In the person with an 80% loss, the remaining vision is 20%. Fifty percent of 20 is 10. The value of 10 is added to the 80%, thus accounting for the 90% reduction in vision noted above.)

In summary, to determine loss of central vision, measure vision at both distance and near, then determine the percentage of loss for each distance. Take the average of the two percentages (and calculate the 50% in the remaining vision if the person is aphakic in only one eye) to determine overall visual function. Remember, the vision in the better eye must have only 20% of vision remaining (or less) in order to qualify for legal blindness. If one (or both) of the two eyes has more than 20% of vision remaining, overall impairment of the visual system can be calculated. (This calculation is presented in the section Impairment of the Visual System.)

## Visual Field Constriction

In terms of determining visual disability based on visual field loss, a single level suprathreshold screening is acceptable. This is generally conducted using the Goldmann perimeter and a III/4e test object. (This is comparable to the old arc perimeter using a 3 mm target at a radius of 330 mm.) If the patient is aphakic, a V/4e test target is used in the Goldmann perimeter or a 6 mm target in the arc perimeter.

Other visual field methods are not considered acceptable for determining visual disability based on visual field constriction at present. Automated perimeters are frequently used in the busy modern ophthalmic office to document visual field loss. There is sufficient variability between the different models in regard to bowl size, target size, target intensity, and background intensity, that the ability to standardize results has been impossible. Likewise, the automated perimeters frequently do not test the visual field beyond 60 degrees, and areas outside of the actual programmed testing area cannot be evaluated. Because of these limitations, automated perimeters have not been considered acceptable in the evaluation of visual field constriction. Automated perimetric results may be used to confirm normal visual fields, however.

Goldmann perimetry provides information that is easily transferred to percentage of lost field. In order to make such calculations, the extent of the normal visual field must be used (see Table A-3 for the extent of the eight principal meridians). The value of each normal meridian is added

**For Distance**

| English | Snellen Notations Metric 6 | Metric 4 | % Loss |
|---------|-----------|----------|--------|
| 20/15 | 6/5 | 4/3 | 0 |
| 20/20 | 6/6 | 4/4 | 0 |
| 20/25 | 6/7.5 | 4/5 | 5 |
| 20/30 | 6/10 | 4/6 | 10 |
| 20/40 | 6/12 | 4/8 | 15 |
| 20/50 | 6/15 | 4/10 | 25 |
| 20/60 | 6/20 | 4/12 | 35 |
| 20/70 | 6/22 | 4/14 | 40 |
| 20/80 | 6/24 | 4/16 | 45 |
| 20/100 | 6/30 | 4/20 | 50 |
| 20/125 | 6/38 | 4/25 | 60 |
| 20/150 | 6/50 | 4/30 | 70 |
| 20/200 | 6/60 | 4/40 | 80 |
| 20/300 | 6/90 | 4/60 | 85 |
| 20/400 | 6/120 | 4/80 | 90 |
| 20/800 | 6/240 | 4/160 | 95 |

**Table A-1a.** Visual acuity notations with corresponding percentages of loss of central vision for distance. (Reprinted with permission from Engelberg AL, ed. *Guides to the Evaluation of Permanent Impairment.* 3rd ed. Philadelphia, Pa: American Medical Association; 1988.)

**For Near**

| Near Snellen Inches | Centimeters | Revised Jaeger Standard | American point-type | % Loss |
|--------|-------------|--------|----------|--------|
| 14/14 | 35/35 | 1 | 3 | 0 |
| 14/18 | 35/45 | 2 | 4 | 0 |
| 14/21 | 35/53 | 3 | 5 | 5 |
| 14/24 | 35/60 | 4 | 6 | 7 |
| 14/28 | 35/70 | 5 | 7 | 10 |
| 14/35 | 35/88 | 6 | 8 | 50 |
| 14/40 | 35/100 | 7 | 9 | 55 |
| 14/45 | 35/113 | 8 | 10 | 60 |
| 14/60 | 35/150 | 9 | 11 | 80 |
| 14/70 | 35/175 | 10 | 12 | 85 |
| 14/80 | 35/200 | 11 | 13 | 87 |
| 14/88 | 35/220 | 12 | 14 | 90 |
| 14/112 | 35/280 | 13 | 21 | 95 |
| 14/140 | 35/350 | 14 | 23 | 98 |

**Table A-1b.** Visual acuity notations with corresponding percentages of loss of central vision for near. (Reprinted with permission from Engelberg AL, ed. *Guides to the Evaluation of Permanent Impairment.* 3rd ed. Philadelphia, Pa: American Medical Association; 1988.)

| Snellen Rating for Distance In Feet | 14/14 | 14/18 | 14/21 | 14/24 | 14/28 | 14/35 | 14/40 | 14/45 | 14/60 | 14/70 | 14/80 | 14/88 | 14/112 | 14/140 |
|------|----|----|----|----|----|----|----|----|----|----|----|----|----|----|
| 20/15 | 0 / 50 | 0 / 50 | 3 / 52 | 4 / 52 | 5 / 53 | 25 / 63 | 27 / 64 | 30 / 65 | 40 / 70 | 43 / 72 | 44 / 72 | 45 / 73 | 48 / 74 | 49 / 75 |
| 20/20 | 0 / 50 | 0 / 50 | 3 / 52 | 4 / 52 | 5 / 53 | 25 / 63 | 27 / 64 | 30 / 65 | 40 / 70 | 43 / 72 | 44 / 72 | 46 / 73 | 48 / 74 | 49 / 75 |
| 20/25 | 3 / 52 | 3 / 52 | 5 / 53 | 6 / 53 | 8 / 54 | 28 / 64 | 30 / 65 | 33 / 67 | 43 / 72 | 45 / 73 | 46 / 73 | 48 / 74 | 50 / 75 | 52 / 76 |
| 20/30 | 5 / 53 | 5 / 53 | 8 / 54 | 9 / 54 | 10 / 55 | 30 / 65 | 32 / 66 | 35 / 68 | 45 / 73 | 48 / 74 | 49 / 74 | 50 / 75 | 53 / 76 | 54 / 77 |
| 20/40 | 8 / 54 | 8 / 54 | 10 / 55 | 11 / 56 | 13 / 57 | 33 / 67 | 35 / 68 | 38 / 69 | 48 / 74 | 50 / 75 | 51 / 76 | 53 / 77 | 55 / 78 | 57 / 79 |
| 20/50 | 13 / 57 | 13 / 57 | 15 / 58 | 16 / 58 | 18 / 59 | 38 / 69 | 40 / 70 | 43 / 72 | 53 / 77 | 55 / 78 | 56 / 78 | 58 / 79 | 60 / 80 | 62 / 81 |
| 20/60 | 16 / 58 | 16 / 58 | 18 / 59 | 20 / 60 | 22 / 61 | 41 / 70 | 44 / 72 | 46 / 73 | 56 / 78 | 59 / 79 | 60 / 80 | 61 / 81 | 64 / 82 | 65 / 83 |
| 20/80 | 20 / 60 | 20 / 60 | 23 / 62 | 24 / 62 | 25 / 63 | 45 / 73 | 47 / 74 | 50 / 75 | 60 / 80 | 63 / 82 | 64 / 82 | 65 / 83 | 68 / 84 | 69 / 85 |
| 20/100 | 25 / 63 | 25 / 63 | 28 / 64 | 29 / 64 | 30 / 65 | 50 / 75 | 52 / 76 | 55 / 78 | 65 / 83 | 68 / 84 | 69 / 84 | 70 / 85 | 73 / 87 | 74 / 87 |
| 20/125 | 30 / 65 | 30 / 65 | 33 / 67 | 34 / 67 | 35 / 68 | 55 / 78 | 57 / 79 | 60 / 80 | 70 / 85 | 73 / 87 | 74 / 87 | 75 / 88 | 78 / 89 | 79 / 90 |
| 20/150 | 34 / 67 | 34 / 67 | 37 / 68 | 38 / 69 | 39 / 70 | 59 / 80 | 61 / 81 | 64 / 82 | 74 / 87 | 77 / 88 | 78 / 89 | 79 / 90 | 82 / 91 | 83 / 92 |
| 20/200 | 40 / 70 | 40 / 70 | 43 / 72 | 44 / 72 | 45 / 73 | 65 / 83 | 67 / 84 | 70 / 85 | 80 / 90 | 83 / 91 | 84 / 92 | 85 / 93 | 88 / 94 | 89 / 95 |
| 20/300 | 43 / 72 | 43 / 72 | 45 / 73 | 46 / 73 | 48 / 74 | 68 / 84 | 70 / 85 | 73 / 87 | 83 / 91 | 85 / 93 | 86 / 93 | 88 / 94 | 90 / 95 | 92 / 96 |
| 20/400 | 45 / 73 | 45 / 73 | 48 / 74 | 49 / 74 | 50 / 75 | 70 / 85 | 72 / 86 | 75 / 88 | 85 / 93 | 88 / 94 | 89 / 94 | 90 / 95 | 93 / 97 | 94 / 97 |
| 20/800 | 48 / 74 | 48 / 74 | 50 / 75 | 51 / 76 | 53 / 77 | 73 / 87 | 75 / 88 | 78 / 89 | 88 / 94 | 90 / 95 | 91 / 96 | 93 / 97 | 95 / 98 | 97 / 99 |

**Table A-2.** Loss of central vision in percentages. Upper figure equals percentage loss of central vision without allowance for monocular aphakia or monocular pseudophakia; lower figure equals percentage loss of central vision with allowance for monocular aphakia or monocular pseudophakia. (Reprinted with permission from Engelberg AL, ed. *Guides to the Evaluation of Permanent Impairment.* 3rd ed. Philadelphia, Pa: American Medical Association; 1988.)

**Table A-3.** Minimal normal extent of monocular visual field from point of fixation. (Reprinted with permission from Engelberg AL, ed. *Guides to the Evaluation of Permanent Impairment.* 3rd ed. Philadelphia, Pa: American Medical Association; 1988.)

| Direction of Vision | Degrees of Field |
| --- | --- |
| Temporally | 85 |
| Down temporally | 85 |
| Direct down | 65 |
| Down nasally | 50 |
| Nasally | 60 |
| Up nasally | 55 |
| Direct up | 45 |
| Up temporally | 55 |
| Total | 500 |

together to obtain the numeric value for a normal visual field. This is compared to the results from the patient's Goldmann visual field test. Let's say that the visual field results reveal a concentric contraction to 30 degrees in each meridian. We must therefore subtract 30 from the normal field values for each meridian (85 − 30 = 55; 85 − 30 = 55; 65 − 30 = 35; 50 − 30 = 20; 60 − 30 = 30; 55−30 = 25; 45 − 30 = 15; 55 − 30 = 25). The differences are added together (in this case, 55 + 55 + 35 + 20 + 30 + 25 + 15 + 25 = 260). This sum of 260 is then divided by 500 (the normal visual field value) in order to determine the percentage of loss. In our example, there is a 52% loss of visual field.

Those with fields of 10 degrees or less in the better eye are considered legally blind. However, a combined visual acuity and visual field loss that does not, in and of itself, qualify the person as legally blind, may be just as disabling. This has been taken into account by those determining visual disability and is referred to as "visual efficiency."

## Visual Efficiency

Visual efficiency is based on the percent of central acuity loss and peripheral field loss in the better eye of a person who does not directly qualify as being legally blind. (Visual efficiency can also be based on visual acuity loss, visual field loss, and restricted ocular mobility. Individuals who are interested in such calculations should review the *Guides to the Evaluation of Permanent Impairment* developed by the AMA.)

Visual efficiency for the better eye can be calculated in the following manner. First, obtain the percentage of central vision loss (see Table A-2) and then calculate central vision efficiency by subtracting percentage loss from 100. Second, obtain the percentage of visual field loss as was described earlier, and then calculate visual field efficiency, also derived by subtracting percentage loss from 100. The differences are then multiplied by 0.01, then multiplied together, and converted to a percentage to reveal overall visual efficiency.

For example, suppose a person has a central vision loss of 56% and a visual field loss of 32%. Fifty-six is subtracted from 100 to leave a difference of 44. Next, 32 is subtracted from 100 to leave a difference of 68. Next, multiply each number by 0.01 (yielding 0.44 and 0.68), and then multiply these two new numbers together. This will produce 0.299. (Remember, both of these numbers represent percentages and should be less than 1, so when multiplied together they should each have a decimal points in front [ie, 0.44 x 0.68 = 0.299]. If the decimal point is not included, the product will be 2,992!) The product is rounded up and multiplied by 100 to get percentage of visual efficiency (0.30 x 100 = 30%). This represents the remaining visual efficiency in this eye. Thus, there is 30% remaining visual efficiency (or a 70% loss of visual efficiency) in the eye. These values may be numerically modified by the presence of other factors such as aphakia (see Table A-2) and diplopia.

## Impairment of the Visual System

There are times when the impairment of the entire visual system may need to be calculated (when visual reduction is less than 80% in both eyes). This is done mathematically, using percentage of loss figures. First, calculate the percentage of loss for each eye, as described above. Second, multiply the value of the better eye by 3 and then add this product to the value from the worse eye. (Unlike the equation above, you do not multiply these numbers by 0.01.) Finally, divide this new sum by 4. This results in a numeric value of impairment of the visual system.

For example, suppose the impairment of the better eye is 30 and the worse eye is 90. Thirty is multiplied by 3, resulting in a product of 90. Now 90 is added to the impairment value of the worse eye, which is 90. This results in a sum of 180, which is then divided by 4. This results in a value of 45. This suggests that there is a 45% impairment in this visual system. The formula looks like this: [(3 x impairment value of better eye) + impairment value of worse eye] ÷ 4.

## Other Visual System Abnormalities Affecting Disability Determination

We have covered several key areas in establishing visual disability, namely loss of central acuity, loss of peripheral vision, or decreased visual efficiency. There are several other factors that are often used in the evaluation of disability. They are ophthalmoplegia and diplopia.

Total bilateral ophthalmoplegia is considered a disabling condition, but because it does not result in a person receiving a label of legal blindness, the individual will not qualify for blind benefits. However, such patients are considered disabled and often qualify for standard disability benefits. Loss of ocular motility can be included in the equation to determine impairment of the visual system. The addition of the percentage of ocular motility loss in the equation may be important and may result in the individual being considered visually disabled.

Severe diplopia can also result in a person being considered disabled. Diplopia within the central 20 degrees results in a 100% impairment of ocular motility. This is due to the fact that central diplopia is considered very disabling, and the only way to effectively eliminate it is by covering one of the eyes.

### Testing Diplopia Via Goldmann Perimetry

Diplopia is measured with a Goldmann perimeter. The patient is seated in the bowl as if visual field testing were to occur. Both eyes are tested simultaneously, and the eyes should be equidistant from the central fixation target. The technician tests each meridian with a III/4e test target. The patient is asked when the target goes from "one" to "two," thus indicating the area where diplopia is present. A standard Goldmann chart is used to indicate the "diplopia field." The technician marks the chart in a manner similar to that when testing the extent of the visual field. Presence of diplopia within the central 30 degrees is considered disabling, whereas peripheral diplopia is generally not considered disabling. The exception to this rule is in the inferior meridians, because of how bothersome diplopia is when reading.

Figure A-1 shows the percent of ocular motility loss due to diplopia within the central 30 degrees. If diplopia is outside of the central 20 degree field and present in more than one meridian, the percentages are added together.

**Figure A-1.** Percentage/loss of ocular motility of one eye in diplopia fields. (Reprinted with permission from Engelberg AL, ed. *Guides to the Evaluation of Permanent Impairment.* 3rd ed. Philadelphia, Pa: American Medical Association; 1988.)

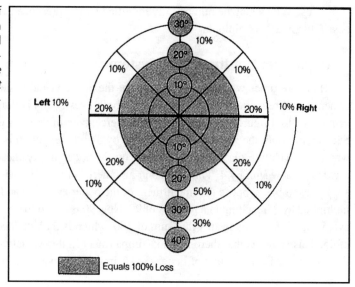

## Other Considerations

There are things besides actual visual acuity that are frequently considered when a person is being evaluated for benefits based on vision loss. Using the requirements set by the Social Security Administration, those individuals whose visual acuity is 20/40 or better in the better eye are not considered visually impaired. Those individuals who have vision of 20/50 or worse may be eligible for some benefits under the Social Security Administration, even when not legally blind.

Let's say that a 63-year-old patient with a long-standing history of hypertension and diabetes mellitus has applied for disability benefits under Social Security. The person has mild diabetic retinopathy resulting in a best corrected vision of 20/60 in both eyes. The requirement for Social Security benefits based on age is 65 years; the requirement for Social Security blind disability benefits is 20/200 after correction in the better eye. The diagnoses of hypertension and diabetes do not necessarily mean that the patient is disabled; however, the combination of these four factors may result in the person receiving standard disability payments under the Social Security Administration. If a person has numerous conditions, even if none of them are disabling, the combination of the conditions may render the individual disabled.

Several other items are also frequently taken into account. The type of occupation the person had prior to the vision loss is frequently considered. How employable the person is now that his or her vision is no longer normal is also considered. The person's age is frequently taken into account as well. If the person is young, he or she may be trained to do other types of work that are not as visually demanding. If the person is older, it may not be cost effective to re-train that individual. These are all questions that are included in the evaluation process for such things as disability payments. If a person is not legally blind, she or he will not be eligible for blind disability payments, which can be higher than standard disability payments in some states. However, the person still may be eligible for some type of compensation based on combined physical and/or mental problems, as well as the other factors just mentioned.

## Proper Documentation

Proper documentation of vision loss has already been covered in part earlier in this section. It must be emphasized how essential such documentation is to the patient. When the physician is making an evaluation, several issues must be covered. First, a medical narrative must be included. This should cover medical conditions, results of most recent laboratory or special tests, assessment of current clinical status, statement of future plans and prognosis, diagnosis, clinical impressions, and expected date of full or partial recovery. Second, an analysis of the findings should be included. This should cover the impact of the medical condition on life activities, a statement indicating the stability of the condition, and a statement indicating whether the person might suffer injury or further impairment by engaging in certain activities. Finally, a comparison of the patient's findings to that of the criteria standards should be included.

It is acceptable to indicate that a person currently meets the requirements of legal blindness, but that the individual might benefit from surgical intervention (such as the removal of a cataract). Although a condition might be surgically remedied, most insurance companies will not force the applicant to have the surgery. Frequently, such individuals are re-evaluated more often than those whose conditions cannot be improved with surgical interventions.

# Universal Precautions

# Introduction

This appendix is designed as a brief overview of universal precautions. It is not designed to provide specific recommendations, only to make you aware of potential issues concerning the universal precautions within the field of eyecare.

Universal precautions have been designed by the Centers for Disease Control (CDC) to ensure that both health care professionals and patients are not inadvertently exposed to harmful antigens such as HIV and hepatitis by means of exposure to blood and other bodily fluids. Moreover, in 1992 the federal Occupational Safety and Health Administration (OSHA) created guidelines for employers which were designed to reduce employees' risk of accidental exposure to bloodborne pathogens. Blood, semen, vaginal and cervical secretions, as well as breast milk are fluids that have high concentrations of HIV (in infected individuals), with the potential of causing transmission of HIV between individuals if exposure occurs. Saliva, tears, perspiration, urine, and feces are considered to have a low infectivity rate for HIV. However, any bodily fluid that either contains blood or is of unknown origin should be considered highly infectious.

In eyecare we are exposed to potentially hazardous body fluids on a very limited basis. Because of this, the American Academy of Ophthalmology (AAO) has designed specific guidelines for the ophthalmic practice which includes federal OSHA guidelines. Any ophthalmologist can obtained these guidelines free of charge through the AAO office in San Francisco, California. Optometrists may obtain a copy through the American Optometric Association (AOA) in Chicago. The guidelines should be adhered to in every practice.

In addition, many states have their own OSHA offices with regulations that may be stricter than federal regulations. Therefore, it is important that each practice contact the state OSHA office to assure that it is in compliance. Fines for non-compliance are very high; however, most state OSHA offices are more than willing to assist a doctor's office in becoming compliant if the office asks for help.

The AAO and AOA guidelines are concerned with reducing the possibility of transmitting bloodborne pathogens such as HIV, as well as ocular surface antigens such as the adenovirus, the cause of EKC (epidemic keratoconjunctivitis). The following discussion will include procedures to protect patients and procedures to protect both office staff and physicians from exposure to bloodborne pathogens and ocular surface antigens.

# Protecting Patients from Exposure

Every patient who comes into an eyecare office expects to be treated with care. This includes the expectation that inadvertent exposure to another patient's ocular infection will not occur. By following these simple precautions with every patient, it is probable that patients coming to the office where you work will not be accidentally exposed to antigens.

It is important that such procedures be performed with and between every patient regardless of the patient volume in the office where you work. First, some individuals may not know their HIV status, so you must assume everyone is HIV positive. (It is impossible to know the HIV status of an individual just by looking at him or her, so do not fall into the trap of thinking that you can tell who is and who is not HIV positive.) HIV has been isolated in the tear film, but at very low concentrations. It is felt that HIV transmission via the tear film is very unlikely, but it is biologically plausible for such transmission to occur. Second, it is most likely that the type of infections transmitted between patients will be the more common ones, such as "pink eye." Contracting the adenovirus results in severe conjunctivitis and is very contagious. Thus, many of the precautions recommended by the CDC, the AAO, and the AOA were made to reduce the risk of EKC transmission between patients.

## Hand Washing

One of the simplest ways to protect patients (and yourself) from inadvertent exposure is by hand washing. If there is a sink in the examination room, wash your hands in front of the patient. This will let the patient know that your hands are clean. Washing with an anti-microbial soap and warm water should be done before and after each patient is examined.

## Eyedrops

Eyedrops can easily become contaminated, potentially housing infective antigens such as the adenovirus. If an eyedropper tip touches the lid, lashes, or conjunctiva of any patient, the dropper should be discarded.

## Protective Wear

Gowns and masks are generally not needed during a routine eye examination in order to protect the patient. Gloves are not generally necessary to protect the patient either, unless the examiner has open sores on his or her hands. Some healthcare workers prefer to wear gloves with all patients; however, that is based primarily on preference. Gloves must be changed between patients if they are worn. An unclean glove can result in transmission of contaminents between patients regardless of whether or not the healthcare provider is well-protected.

It is recommended that gloves be worn when examining a patient with a "red" eye. It must also be remembered that gloves are not a substitute for hand washing, and that hands should be washed after the removal of gloves. Gloves cannot be left on and washed between patients: they were designed for single use only.

## Disinfection of Equipment

Disinfecting equipment between patients is essential. The CDC recommends a 1:10 bleach to water solution to inactivate HIV, hepatitis, herpes simplex, and the adenovirus. Usually an instrument is soaked in the solution for 5 minutes, followed by a sterile water rinse for several minutes. (Although the use of tap water is frequently mentioned in precautionary guidelines, the CDC does not recommend its use, as using tap water will introduce the clean instrument to the flora and fauna found in the local water supply.)

Alternately, a 3% hydrogen peroxide solution can be used for a 5-minute soak with a sterile water rinse to follow. The hydrogen peroxide solution must be changed twice daily.

Finally, the AAO has suggested that isopropyl alcohol can be used to disinfect instruments in most instances. (Alcohol does not require a sterile water rinse as it dries very quickly.) The CDC reports that isopropyl alcohol does not effectively kill all of the adenoviruses (unlike the bleach solution), therefore the CDC does not recommend the use of alcohol. However, the vigorous wiping of instruments for 5 minutes with isopropyl alcohol can be used to inactivate HIV, hepatitis viruses, herpes simplex, and most, but not all, of the adenoviruses. (Both the AAO and the AOA guidelines include 70% isopropyl alcohol as a disinfectant for equipment such as tonometer tips.) When isopropyl alcohol is used, the instrument should be allowed to dry for at least 1 to 2 minutes before it is used on another patient. Disinfection with a 1:10 bleach solution would still be essential after an instrument has been used on any patient with a suspected adenovirus infection.

We must remember that no disinfection solution is perfect, each has its pluses and minuses. The 1:10 bleach solution kills virtually all infectious agents, but can be harmful to certain instruments and the cornea. It dries slowly, and instruments cleaned with this solution must be rinsed in sterile water or saline after disinfection. Build up of bleach deposits has been seen in tonometer tips, and these build-ups can cause damage in eyes that have recently undergone refractive surgery.[1]

Hydrogen peroxide (3%) is also an excellent surface disinfectant, but it too can cause damage to the cornea and certain instruments, and dries very slowly. The solution needs to be changed at least twice daily and instruments cleaned with 3% hydrogen peroxide must be rinsed as well.

Seventy percent isopropyl alcohol is an excellent surface disinfectant, but is less effective. It dries quickly, and if an instrument is allowed to dry for 10 to 15 minutes, rinsing is not always necessary (unless there are areas on the instrument where the alcohol can pool).

Finally, sterilizing solutions containing 2% glutaraldehyde have been used to disinfect many ophthalmic instruments. This solution causes little damage to instruments but is very toxic to humans. Some state OSHAs have restricted its use in a clinical setting as a result of its toxicity. Care must be taken when choosing the disinfection solution to clean specific instruments and devices. Seeking advice on specific instrument disinfection is recommended.

Most instrument companies have developed appropriate methods for instrument disinfection. These methods are generally based on AAO or CDC recommendations and the tolerance of the instrument for a particular disinfecting agent. Individuals should check their manuals or contact the company directly to find out the best disinfection procedure. These procedures may have changed over the years, and newer instruments may need to be disinfected differently from older models of the same instrument.

## Ultrasound Instrumentation

For ultrasound probes, different companies have different disinfection policies based on the probe material and the permeability of the membranous tip. Most hard tipped A-scan probes can be disinfected with either 1:10 bleach solution, 3% hydrogen peroxide, or 70% isopropyl alcohol. The applanating surface and adjacent 3 mm of the probe should be immersed in the solution for 5 minutes, rinsed in sterile water (manufacturers frequently suggest tap water) and allowed to air dry.

B-scan probes have flexible membranes, and most manufacturers do not recommend the use of 70% isopropyl alcohol because this can dry out the membrane. Soaking the probe, as described above, in either 3% hydrogen peroxide or a 1:10 bleach solution is recommended by many (but not all) manufacturers.

Scleral shells for immersion ultrasonography should be rinsed thoroughly after use on a patient to remove the methylcellulose. Once rinsed, the shell can be either vigorously wiped with a 70% isopropyl alcohol pad, or soaked in a 3% hydrogen peroxide solution for 5 minutes. If the shell has been soaked in peroxide, it must be soaked in sterile saline for 5 minutes, air dried, and put away.

## Laser, Diagnostic, and Acrylic Surgical Lenses

These lenses are very delicate and need to be properly handled. As soon as the lens is removed from the patient's eye it should be thoroughly rinsed under tap water. For disinfection, the manufacturer suggests soaking the lenses in a 2% glutaraldehyde solution for 20 minutes, or a 1:10 bleach solution for 10 minutes. The lenses cannot be soaked for any longer than this amount of time or damage can occur. The lenses must be rinsed thoroughly and dried and put away in dry storage.

### Burian-Allen Contact Lens Electrodes for ERG Testing

Rinse the contact lens thoroughly in tap water immediately after removing it from the patient's eye. To disinfect the lens, the manufacturer recommends soaking the lens in a 1:10 bleach solution for 5 minutes (and no longer) followed by a thorough rinsing in sterile water. Soaking the lenses longer than 5 minutes or in a solution stronger than 1:10 can cause corrosion to the delicate wires on the electrode. The manufacturer recommends a 20-minute soak in a 2% glutaraldehyde solution and reports that no damage occurred to the lens after a 4-day soak in this solution. Thoroughly rinse the lens in sterile water after the 20-minute soak. Three percent hydrogen peroxide causes damage to the lens and is not recommended.

### Contact Lenses

Trial contact lenses must be disinfected between patients. For gas permeable or hard contact lenses, disinfectants that contain hydrogen peroxide or chlorhexidene will inactive potential antigens. Disinfection of soft contact lens with either hydrogen peroxide or heat systems is adequate.

### Other Surfaces

Other surfaces such as slit lamps, may need to be disinfected as well. HIV is a very fragile virus and does not live long outside of the human body. Adenoviruses are not fragile and live on surfaces for quite some time. Therefore, if a patient with suspected EKC has been seen in the office, other surfaces (such as counters, slit lamp, and slit lamp stand) will need to be wiped down with either a 1:10 bleach solution or a hospital disinfectant. Isopropyl alcohol should probably not be used, as several of the adenovirus are not deactivated by alcohol. Wiping slit lamp surfaces with alcohol between patients is acceptable if the preceding patient did not have conjunctivitis. Any conjunctivitis should be treated as an adenovirus infection, to be on the safe side.

## Protecting Staff and Physicians from Exposure

Protecting staff and physicians from possible exposure is an equally important task. According to OSHA it is the responsibility of the employer (be it the physician or clinic) to keep the staff protected from possible exposure to bloodborne pathogens. These precautions should be used to protect every healthcare worker who comes in contact with patients.

In order to be in compliance with OSHA regulations, employers of healthcare workers who come in contact with patients and who may be at risk for exposure to bloodborne pathogens must set up policies to reduce the risk of exposure to bloodborne pathogens. The policies must address the possible risk of occupational exposure and ways by which risk of exposure can be substantially reduced or eliminated. Employees must go through training on exposure-reduction procedures, and the training must be documented in the employee's employment records. The trainer's qualifications must be indicated as well as the information that was covered in the training session. Finally, all employees who are at risk of exposure (through contact with needles, blood, or blood products) must receive hepatitis B vaccinations (provided at the employer's expense) or sign a declination statement which states that the individual has been given the opportunity to receive the vaccination but has declined the offer.

Since tears are not considered to be infectious bodily fluids, many of the OSHA preventive measures are unnecessary; however, any fluid that contains blood or is of unknown origin must be considered infectious. Following certain hygienic procedures during routine eye examinations will greatly reduce the risk of exposure.

## Hand Washing

Hand washing between patients is an effective means by which to reduce possible exposure to many pathogens that are encountered in the eyecare setting. Hands should be dried with clean paper towels, and nails should be kept short and clean.

## Gloves

Although individuals within an eyecare setting may be at fairly low risk for occupational exposure, gloves should be available in each exam room. This will reduce the potential for accidental exposure in the event that gloves are needed and not immediately available. Gloves used for examination purposes (where direct contact with open skin is unlikely) and fluorescein angiograms (or other injections) need not be sterile. However, any minor surgery will need to be conducted with sterile gloves. Gloves should never be used in substitution for hand washing, and should only be used once. The same pair of gloves should never be used between patients. These items must be provided to each employee at no cost to the employee.

## Protective Wear

In routine eye examinations, gowns, masks, and protective eye wear are not necessary. However, the healthcare worker must wear protective eye wear during any procedure in which blood or blood-filled fluids may splash. Judgment must be used about protective clothing and eyewear when minor surgery is performed in the office. When photorefractive keratectomy procedures are performed, gloves, gowns, masks, and protective eyewear should be worn. This is because viruses can become air-borne during the procedure, thus increasing the risk of potential exposure. All protective wear must be provided to employees at no cost to the employee.

## Handling of Tissue

The examiner will often come into contact with tissue, including mucous membranes, during an eye examination. Gloves can be worn to reduce potential exposure, or individuals can adopt the "no-touch" technique (ungloved) to reduce the risk of exposure. In the "no-touch" technique, cotton swabs (or some similar items) are used to retract the lid during the examination. Finger cots (look like the finger ends of rubber gloves, without the hand part) can also be used instead of full gloves. In this way, the examiner does not have to wear gloves, but does not come in direct contact with the tissues of the patient. Any blood that is drawn from a patient or any culture that is made should be considered contaminated and handled with extreme caution. All blood and tissue must be marked with appropriate labels in order to warn others that the material is potentially contaminated.

## Handling of Sharp Instruments

The CDC has specific recommendations for the handling of sharp instruments ("sharps"), which includes scalpel blades and needles. In general, extreme caution should be used for every aspect of handling (including during the procedure, after the procedure, and when cleaning instruments) and instrument disposal. In general, used sharp instruments are considered hazardous waste and should be handled using a "no-touch" technique in order to reduce inadvertent exposure. This means that needles should not be re-capped and should only be placed in a sharps container. The sharps containers are made of heavy plastic (generally red color-coded) that is not easily punctured. Sharp items can be easily placed inside the sharps container, but the opening does not allow for easy removal. Any sharp, disposable item must be placed in a sharps container, which should be easily accessible in every exam room. Disposal of full containers must be done in accordance with state or local ordinances.

## Handling of Contaminated Waste

In addition to sharp objects that may be contaminated, other items such as surgical drapes may be contaminated with blood and body fluids. If there is little blood on a drape that was used during a surgical procedure, it does not need to be considered hazardous waste. In the event that the drape is quite bloody, it must be disposed of in an orange bag marked with the universal symbol for biologic hazard (Figure B-1). If the drape or sheet is wringing wet from blood or unknown bodily fluids (very unlikely in an eyecare setting) it must be placed in a leak-proof container or bag.

## Labeling

Labeling is an important means of communicating to others that the enclosed item is a biohazardous waste and possibly contaminated. The use of either orange bags with the biohazard insignia or the "red container" are acceptable means by which to indicate and dispose of hazardous materials. Sharp items that are disposable or reusable must be placed in a red container. Also, containers used for storage or transportation of blood, blood products, specimens, or waste must be appropriately labeled. Contaminated equipment in need of servicing or soiled laundry must also be labeled. Finally, refrigerators that contain specimens or blood products must be labeled. Failure to label appropriately can result in serious fines from OSHA.

## Surgery

Using universal precautions during surgery means that linen and instruments must be handled and discarded in a specific way to reduce the possibility of exposure. Anyone performing or assisting in surgery should use care not to come in direct contact with sharp objects such as needles or scalpels. Needle holders and forceps should be used to touch sharp instruments. In instances where the sharp instrument must be handled, the individual should touch only the handle of the instrument. Accidental puncture of the glove or skin should be avoided at all costs. In the event that the skin is accidentally punctured during surgery, the individual should stop participating in surgery (when possible). The wound should be soaked in an antiseptic for 5 minutes and then dressed in a usual fashion. If the person is vital to the surgery, the individual can re-glove and continue to participate in the procedure only if the wound is no longer weeping.

# Exposure

Any individual is considered to have been exposed to bloodborne pathogens if a needle stick, cut, or puncture with a used or contaminated item occurs. Exposure also occurs if blood or body

**Figure B-1.** This biohazardous symbol must be used on all biohazardous materials and waste. (Photograph by Nilo Davila.)

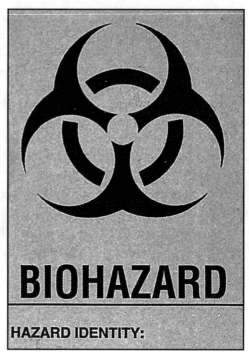

fluids of unknown origin splash onto mucous membranes or maintain prolonged cutaneous contact. There are several procedures that must be followed subsequent to such exposure.

First, the source (patient) should be notified of the healthcare worker's exposure and then tested for HIV antibodies after informed consent has been obtained. In the event the source patient is unwilling to undergo the test, is HIV positive, or has been diagnosed with AIDS, the exposed healthcare worker should seek medical advice. In many instances, the healthcare worker will be treated prophylactically.

Second, in most instances the healthcare worker will be tested for HIV antibodies and counseled on the signs and symptoms that might indicate HIV seroconversion. Such symptoms include fever, flu-like symptoms, swollen lymph nodes, and rash; these can occur as many as 12 weeks after exposure.

Any healthcare worker who is HIV negative at first testing should be tested again at 6 weeks after exposure. If he or she is still HIV negative, a repeat test should be run 6 months after exposure.

If the source is HIV positive, the exposed employee will require counseling in how to reduce the possibility of inadvertently exposing other individuals. In the event that the source person is HIV negative and at low risk for acquiring HIV, no further intervention with the healthcare worker is necessary. If the source person is HIV negative, but is considered to be at high risk for HIV infection, the healthcare worker is initially treated as if exposed to the blood of a person who is HIV positive. The healthcare worker is told to seek medical advice and is tested for HIV at 6 weeks and then again at 6 months. After 6 month's time, if seroconversion did not take place, the healthcare worker is presumed to be HIV free.

The incident is documented and all information pertaining to this matter is maintained in the healthcare worker's personnel file.

In the event that a patient is inadvertently exposed to the blood of another patient or a healthcare worker, a similar procedure as outlined above should be followed.

## Record Keeping

Records must be kept on all employees in reference to exposure, hepatitis B vaccination status, and training. In the event that an employee has been exposed to potential bloodborne pathogens, that information must be kept in the employee's record. The information must include the employee's name and social security number, hepatitis B vaccination status, results of post-exposure medical examinations and testing, attending doctor's written professional opinion, and a copy of the information provided to the exposed individual. This information must be kept confidentially in the personnel file for the entire time of employment plus an additional 30 years. In the event that the individual has declined a hepatitis B vaccination, the signed letter of declination must also be included in the file.

Records regarding training in universal precautions and exposure prevention must also be included in the person's file. Such information must include training dates, content of training session, name and qualifications of trainer(s), and name and job title of those in attendance.

# Reference

1. Maldonado MJ. Corneal epithelial alterations resulting from use of chlorine-disinfected contact tonometer after myopic photorefractive keratectomy. *Ophthalmology.* 1998;105:1546-1549.

# Index

# For your information

This book and many others on numerous different topics are available from SLACK Incorporated. For further information or a copy of our latest catalog, contact us at:

**Professional Book Division**
**SLACK Incorporated**
**6900 Grove Road**
**Thorofare, NJ 08086 USA**
**Telephone: 1-609-848-1000, 1-856-848-100**
**1-800-257-8290**
**Fax: 1-609-853-5991, 1-856-853-5991**
**E-mail: orders@slackinc.com**
**WWW: http://www.slackinc.com**

We accept most major credit cards and checks or money orders in US dollars drawn on a US bank. Most orders are shipped within 72 hours.

Contact us for information on recent releases, forthcoming titles, and bestsellers. If you have a comment about this title or see a need for a new book, direct your correspondence to the Editorial Director at the above address.

If you are an instructor, we can be reached at the address listed above or on the Internet at *educomps@slackinc.com* for specific needs.

Thank you for your interest and we hope you found this work beneficial.